Covid – an Alternative Inquiry

PETER LANG
PROMPT

PETER LANG
Lausanne - Berlin - Bruxelles - Chennai - New York - Oxford

David Williams

Covid – an Alternative Inquiry

Putting Health at the Heart of a Green Recovery Strategy

PETER LANG

Lausanne - Berlin - Bruxelles - Chennai - New York - Oxford

Bibliographic information published by the Deutsche Nationalbibliothek. The German National Library lists this publication in the German National Bibliography; detailed bibliographic data is available on the Internet at http://dnb.d-nb.de.

A catalogue record for this book is available from the British Library.

Library of Congress Control Number: 2023037406

ISBN 978-1-80374-284-7 (print)
ISBN 978-1-80374-292-2 (ePDF)
ISBN 978-1-80374-293-9 (ePub)
DOI 10.3726/b21150

© 2023 Peter Lang Group AG, Lausanne
Published by Peter Lang Ltd, Oxford, United Kingdom
info@peterlang.com - www.peterlang.com

David Williams has asserted his right under the Copyright, Designs and Patents Act, 1988, to be identified as Author of this Work.

All rights reserved.
All parts of this publication are protected by copyright.
Any utilisation outside the strict limits of the copyright law, without the permission of the publisher, is forbidden and liable to prosecution. This applies in particular to reproductions, translations, microfilming, and storage and processing in electronic retrieval systems.

This publication has been peer reviewed.

Contents

List of tables — vii

Introduction — 1

CHAPTER 1
Using sound science responsibly — 5

CHAPTER 2
Living within the planet's environmental limits — 29

CHAPTER 3
Achieving a sustainable economy — 55

CHAPTER 4
Ensuring a strong, healthy and just society — 79

CHAPTER 5
Promoting good governance — 101

Conclusion — 129

Index — 133

Tables

Table 1.	World statistics on Covid-19; 21/1/2022	5
Table 2.	Covid traffic in Great Britain as percentage of pre-Covid levels	33
Table 3.	Passenger transport in Great Britain, 1979–2019	33
Table 4.	European rail passenger traffic, 1900–2003	40
Table 5.	European rail freight traffic ('000 tonnes), 1900–2003	42
Table 6.	British bus services and passenger trips, 1985/6–2008/9	45
Table 7.	Annual social transport urban trips by nation, 1983–2008	49
Table 8.	£220 million Community Renewal Fund in England, 2022	82
Table 9.	Tax spending on education, health and housing 1982/3–2018/9 as percentage of GDP	97
Table 10.	UK government tax income £m, 2007/8	118

Introduction

This book provides a British agenda for action as we recover from Covid. It differs from the official UK Public Inquiry in three important respects.

The official inquiry will focus on our preparedness before Covid struck, how the government managed the pandemic, how the health services and private sector agents performed, and the effectiveness of public messaging – before defining a strategy that better prepares us for any future pandemic. That is very specific.

This inquiry looks wider. As Covid spread through society, it often revealed how we mismanaged all public services, not just health. This anecdotal evidence of Covid is vital if we are to learn from the light it shed on this wider landscape. As an analogy, instead of a Public Inquiry's surgical dissection under the microscope, this inquiry looks at the broader social and political horizon revealed by a telescope.

Second, the official inquiry is essentially backward-looking, reviewing what went wrong. This inquiry looks forward to how we should recover. The EU set the challenge. "Building the resilience of our health systems and promoting a green recovery has never been so urgent" (*Health at a Glance: Europe 2020*). While Covid confirmed how vulnerable our health service is, the major issue is how to achieve a green recovery. Too often during Covid, the government's political priorities conflicted with sustainable principles.

This requires immediate action, and cannot wait at least three years before the official inquiry completes its vital democratic task. This alternative inquiry addresses those conflicts now, using the UK government's own sustainable development strategy, *Securing the Future* (2011). This contains 'five guiding principles', which head the following five chapters. Each chapter defines a generic 'health' issue, with reference to specific public services.

1. 'Using sound science responsibly' looks at personal well-being and our health services.
2. 'Living within the planet's environmental limits' discusses environmental health in relation to transport and household emissions.
3. To 'achieve a sustainable economy' focusses on strengthening local economies that mix private and public enterprise, exemplified with farming.
4. To 'ensure a strong, healthy and just society' for social health means reducing gross wealth and health inequalities, illustrated by education and housing; and
5. "Promoting good governance' requires expertise, integrity, efficiency and tax reform for a healthy democracy.

As an indication of government commitment, these five principles were included in the *NPPF (National Planning Policy Framework)* 2012, but not in two subsequent editions. During Covid (coming after ten years of austerity and complicated by Brexit), all-too-often these guiding principles were either ignored or contradicted. We need to identify these failures so that, as we emerge from Covid, we can hold the government to its own guiding principles for a more sustainable future in all walks of public life.

This is not an academic book. It is an agenda – or prompt – for sustainable action with three other strategic themes:

- public health in all its aspects; not just personal well-being but also environmental protection, economic resilience and social fairness;
- local devolution, each chapter concluding with the scope for councils to deliver more public services like health, transport, education and housing; and
- political balance between libertarian values and social equity: between, for example, 'market demand' and human rights, motorists' convenience and transport efficiency, private wealth and social health, 'the politics of change' and the need for continuity. This, of course, is the stuff of politics.

Three final points by way of introduction. This Covid inquiry is based largely on the British experience, with international comparisons where available. The occasional lapses into 'we' and 'our' simply refer to UK citizens and its government. Foreign readers might like to know how another nation coped, but also how a pragmatic, 'fair-minded' democracy has become increasingly incompetent and intolerant under successive governments.

Second, the text relies heavily on articles since March 2020 from *The Observer*, *Private Eye* and *Wikipedia*, the EU and OECD *Health at a Glance: Europe 2020*, various BBC documentaries, notably *Hospital*, the last (lamented) print edition of the ONS *Annual Abstract of Statistics* (2010), and my book *Civilizing Cities*.

Finally, some may find my choice of words occasionally flippant. I can only plead that 'foodshed', for example, is more accurate than 'supermarket', 'mega-corp' simpler than 'multi-national corporation', 'exoskeleton' more suggestive of the anti-social nature of cars, and the 'Bankers' Crash' of 2008 more honest.

CHAPTER 1

Using sound science responsibly

Personal health and Covid

Health is defined by the World Health Organization (WHO) as "a state of complete physical, mental and social well-being and not merely the absence of disease or infirmity." Covid seriously affected all three states of well-being.

With so many variables, and so few politicians who understand science, it is difficult to 'measure' the health of a nation. Covid, however, does provide a crude measure of how each nation coped with the pandemic, the capacity of their health services and the underlying health of their population.

Table 1. World statistics on Covid-19; 21/1/2022

Nation	Cases	Deaths	Cases/ Deaths per 1 million population	% Deaths/ Cases		Xs Death/ 1 million population*
				Aug-20	Jan-22	
1 US	70,544,862	883,903	211,203/ 2,646	2.6	1.3	3,140
3 Brazil	23,588,921	622,251	109,765/ 2,895	2.8	2.6	3,140
4 UK	15,709,059	153,490	229,533/2,243	2.7	1	2,170
5 France	15,600,647	128,114	238,186/1,956	1.9	0.8	1,370
6 Russia	10,987,774	324,752	75,242/2,224	1.7	3	7,420

8 Italy	9,597,362	142,963	159,097/2,370	7.1	1.5	2,890
9 Spain	8,834,363	91,599	188,838/1,958	3.1	1	2,410
10 Germany	8,475,578	117,122	100,660/1,391	2.3	1.4	1,720
18 N'lands	3,778,287	21,200	219,748/1,233	2.4	0.6	1,860
25 Belgium	2,642,761	28,759	226,499/2,465	3.5	1.1	1,990
28 Portugal	2,118,125	19,496	208,671/1,921	1.9	1.1	2,430
31 Australia	2,090,810	2,984	80,543/115	3.3	0.1	-140
32 Japan	2,017,351	18,469	16,028/147	1.8	0.9	150
35 Switz'land	1,871,340	12,675	213,799/1,448	2	0.7	1,350
36 Sweden	1,748,005	15,639	174,954/1,534	5.3	0.7	1,150
37 Greece	1,762,870	22,476	170,424/2,173	1.9	1.3	1,720
40 Austria	1,503,668	13,956	165,490/1,536	1.2	0.9	1,740
43 Denmark	1,270,566	3,371	218,166/613	1.7	0.3	440
45 Ireland	1,127,951	6,087	224,542/1,212	3.4	0.5	560
59 S Korea	719,269	6,501	14,011/127	1.8	0.9	0
69 Norway	571,655	1,413	104,183/258	1.6	0.2	290
78 Finland	426,826	1,815	76,849/327	2.4	0.4	690
118 China	105,484	4,636	73/3	5	4.1	na
171 N Zealand	15,401	52	3,079/10	1.3	0.3	-530

Source: www:worldometers.info
The Economist

All such statistics have anomalies, but some tentative conclusions emerge from Table 1.

Some nations may have under-reported Covid-related deaths, just as some Communist and Catholic nations may still under-report suicides. China is clearly an outlier, with minimal cases and deaths per million, despite being the source of the pandemic. This suggests vigorous control of data or people, or both. It may also explain the highest mortality rate of those infected – more than one in 25 – with little improvement in treatment over the period. (Ominously, its excess death rates from the last column compared with the previous five years are not available!)

Under-reporting may also explain the odd statistics for Russia. With its low infection rate, it recorded the highest excess mortality rate over the previous five years, reflecting both Covid and non-Covid-related deaths.

By contrast, the political response of the US and Brazil was largely to brazen it out. This 'macho' approach resulted in the highest excess death rates after Russia. Curiously, all four nations shared a similar 'fascist' approach, here meaning a strident nationalism defined by, and largely identified with, a strong leader.

More democratic nations, like Denmark, Japan, South Korea and New Zealand, focussed on protecting citizens rather than personal egos. It may be significant that two prime ministers and one health minister were women – in Denmark, New Zealand and South Korea. The contrast between South Korea and the US is instructive. Not only was South Korea well-prepared and decisive in its border controls and test and tracking (T&T). Its citizens also showed commendable social responsibility by allowing the government to track their movements via their mobile phones. This would have been unacceptable in the strongly libertarian US.

Effective early border controls were a major factor in Japan, New Zealand and South Korea. In Europe, this was a major challenge with its myriad entry points and internal freedom of movement. And most of Europe was unprepared. Italy and Spain especially were caught by the initial wave, from which they struggled to gain control. Belgium also suffered because it lacked a government for those crucial early weeks before the several Flemish and Walloon parties formed a coalition.

Socio-geographic factors also affected infection rates. Scandinavia, with its cooler climate, lower densities and possibly lower levels of social behaviour, had lower infection rates compared with the dense urban populations and street markets in the warm Mediterranean basin. Within Scandinavia, Sweden had the highest infection rates, which were not much lower than the UK or US. However, it controlled Covid much more effectively with clear public messaging, stressing the need for social distancing, wearing masks and working from home where possible, so its mortality rate was significantly lower. Treating citizens as responsible adults was not the British approach.

Urban density is another factor. Low-density suburbs may reduce the spread of any virus as they also reduce social behaviour. Dense neighbourhoods do not cause pandemics, but facilitate their spread, particularly among the poor. The wealthy in their spacious homes, being less sociable, survived in some of the densest neighbourhoods. By contrast, ordinary people are more gregarious, and overcrowding is a symptom of acute poverty. If everybody enjoyed 'a living wage' and access to social housing, overcrowding would only remain a short-term expedient in typical family life cycles.

High-density cities are the crucial theatre for healthy economic, social and family life. Today's plagues, involving the transfer of disease from 'lower' animals to humans, are caused by reckless human activities, see next chapter. While cities do facilitate the rare pandemics, we can mitigate their impact. Some, however, will misconstrue this impact of density, and release an altogether different, more virulent virus. We must prevent British plagues of builders and developers forever destroying existing neighbourhoods and building new suburbs, encouraged by zero VAT, compulsory purchase, ambitious architects, utopian planners and credulous (or corrupt) politicians. Buildings and neighbourhoods should last centuries rather than decades, see Chapters 3 and 4.

Covid mortality rates also reflect levels of personal health and fitness. While British and Dutch infection rates were similar, our mortality rate was nearly 60 per cent higher. If diets are similar, then the Dutch must be fitter – due largely to their walking and cycling to work. British motorists average 10,000 miles a year, waste up to three years of life sitting in their exoskeletons and poison citizens with their emissions (Chapter 2).

Our political response

Every nation developed its own response. The UK government was plagued by inappropriate dogma, centralized control and fatal dithering – disguised under a Churchillian 'bunker' mode. During war, rigid central control and secrecy are paramount. During a pandemic, sharing information and involving all relevant agencies are paramount.

The first problem was Britain's 'unpreparedness'. In 2011, we had a 'flu pandemic preparedness strategy' which was highly rated by WHO. In 2016, however, a three-day trial (Exercise Cygnus) involving all relevant health agencies revealed just how ill-prepared we were, despite the strategy. We lacked surge capacity in hospitals, adequate PPE and ventilators, a clear decision-making process and effective public messaging. These failings, revealed when Covid struck, were compounded by inadequate border controls and monitoring systems.

Yet the flu strategy and Exercise Cygnus were never published, ostensibly because they might lead to panic among the public. More likely, they exposed the damage caused by Osborne's austerity cuts to public spending, even as he cut taxes for corporations and the wealthy.

Pandemic risks, accurately forecast by various government studies, were completely ignored (*British Medical Journal*, 11/12/21). How did this happen? Basically, the UK government knew – or should have known – how ill-prepared we were for any pandemic. When Covid struck, we all found out.

It gets worse. Only recently did a dedicated pursuer of the truth, NHS consultant Moosa Qureshi, unearth (under Freedom of Information) several other pandemic exercises prepared by Public Health England (PHE). One of these, Exercise Alice, was for MERS, a more relevant pandemic than flu. Such secrecy has no justification.

Occasionally, the government worsened the situation. For example, after the Bankers' Crash in 2008, we actually *reduced* the number of hospital beds by a further 7,000. The NHS was already struggling. Where were the media? When Covid patients quickly filled intensive care beds, cancellations of non-urgent and most urgent non-Covid operations could no longer be ignored. This increased non-Covid deaths, and a backlog that hospitals will long struggle to reduce.

Having outsourced the purchase and distribution of PPE, much was simply unusable. And after Brexit, the government knew that we would need about 30,000 more customs officers to cope with the expected border chaos, but did nothing for three years. Covid compounded that chaos.

The initial response was that this was simply another flu variant – we should brazen it out and develop 'herd immunity'. When it became clear how virulent Covid was, with deaths rising alarmingly, the government relied (in varying degrees) on advice from SAGE, the scientific advisory group for emergencies with 40 experts. This may be too many, leading either to factions 'fighting corners', or under intense pressure, all succumbing to a messy 'group think'. Nor were the SAGE findings made public. Control of data may be the politicians' *modus operandi,* but it contradicts both the nature of scientific speculation and the spirit of democracy. Most seriously, perhaps, SAGE had no public health expert (although 'special advisor' Dominic Cummings was thought fit to attend the meetings). So an 'Alternative Sage' was set up, with more relevant experts, with the aim of being open with all its discussions and findings.

In any event, government control of all data and policy revealed at least four serious faults. First, early mortality data was based solely on daily deaths in hospitals, 'because it's accurate and quick'. It was not until 28th April that deaths at home and in care homes were included. This under-reporting of deaths delayed the first lockdown. While some nations ordered lockdowns when total Covid deaths exceeded 1,000, Britain was already approaching *1,000 deaths a day* before our first lockdown. Were government ministers unaware of the situation in our care homes, which then accounted for a third of all deaths? It beggars belief that council registrars, in contact with local hospitals, care homes and coroners, could not have provided accurate daily statistics for their areas.

Equally flawed was public messaging. Having disbanded the civil service 'public information unit', the government outsourced it to advertisers, who love short messages. The first said "Stay home. Protect the NHS. Save lives". So, many people stayed home when they needed medical attention, and died there. Almost as culpable, families and friends were not allowed socially-distanced recreation in parks and gardens, where exercise and fresh air would be healthier than being cooped up indoors. The second public message, "Stay alert. Control the virus. Save lives" was clever but confusing. South Korea, New Zealand and Scandinavia provided much more effective public information.

Third, when South Korea set up their effective Test and Trace (T&T) system, most nations followed suit. Sweden, though more 'relaxed' than the UK in its response to Covid, was better at public messaging, and set up an effective T&T system. With no lockdowns, Covid deaths in Sweden were higher than the rest of Scandinavia, but much lower than the UK. We would have a 'world-beating' privatized T&T system in place by 1st June. This was impossible. With no effective border controls to test and isolate arrivals, Covid was already rampant, and PHE (Public Health England) was overwhelmed in tracking those infected. The private companies only 'got to grips' with T&T when infections were declining. But even then, the system still failed to test, trace and isolate sufficient numbers – resulting in two further lockdowns. This failure needs to be explained.

Some also queried T&T. According to Maggie Rae, president of the Faculty of Public Health: "Test and trace is not cost-effective and it's not an early warning system... Testing doesn't tell us how many people have got the virus, just those who have come forward for a test. Wastewater could give you a very good sense of unknown infections that you can then track." (*Observer*, 7/3/21) Was this option considered? We used it to detect outbreaks of polio, and for Covid it was used, apparently, in Australia and Barcelona.

However, in the first three months, local public health teams did perhaps 75 per cent of the T&T in their areas, phoning those infected, following up contacts by knocking on doors, and advising residents and whole streets how to control the spread of infection. The success of Wiltshire public health in dealing with the Russian Novichok poisoning, which could have killed thousands of Salisbury residents, demonstrated the value of rapid response by local experts. Instead, we relied on a few large test sites, national call centres and a late, underperforming tracing App. (P. 70/2 discusses the T&T system further.)

This confirms the fourth fault. Central policy was badly co-ordinated. Local authorities were merely told what to do, usually with only 24 hours' notice and often against their own judgement. This ignored a whole tier of public health expertise and local infrastructure able to implement effective measures quickly. While Northern Ireland, Scotland and Wales have delegated powers, large city regions do not. So when the government relaxed the first lockdown for England, many regions, 'behind the curve' of the southeast, still had rising infections and were not ready to relax their lockdown. In Greater Manchester, the 38 council leaders and sitting MPs (of all parties) agreed that government control was inept and that, given the necessary funds and powers, they could have responded locally more quickly and controlled Covid more effectively.

Later, the government did decide on local exceptions. When Leicester city council was told to impose an emergency lockdown, it was only informed the day before it was to be implemented on 29th June 2021.

At base, the government did little to protect our care homes, and was unable to ease our overcrowded hospitals. Although the army promptly delivered ten Nightingale hospitals to take recovering Covid patients and free up hospital beds, costing about £500 million, they were as promptly mothballed. With already-understaffed hospitals being further depleted by staff infections, there were no spare nurses. Perhaps the government foresaw the problem but thought it better to 'spaff money up the wall' and create headlines.

There was one British success in the first year of Covid. The Oxford vaccine was largely developed with government research funds through the university Jenner Institute. Kate Bingham (a business leader married to a Conservative MP and put in charge of the vaccine programme) helped negotiate a partnership between the Oxford labs and Astra-Zeneca to manufacture and distribute the vaccine at cost rather than with a commercial price based on demand. Thus the Oxford-AZ jab cost about £3 rather than £30+ for the Pfizer jab. However, this success suffered some skewed public messaging.

- Some national judgements were clouded. As frequently happens with vaccine trials, one or two bad reactions pause any trial for a week or two. In the US, this pause extended over four months, during which time their Pfizer and Moderna vaccines received approval. And in Europe, both President Macron and Chancellor Merkel publicly dismissed the Oxford-AZ vaccine.

- Internationally, it played an important role in controlling the pandemic. COVAX, a French, WHO and EU initiative from April 2020, aimed to distribute Covid vaccines to poorer nations. By February 2021, COVAX forecast a distribution of 320 million doses, 318.8 million of them the Oxford-AZ vaccine. Delivering an effective vaccine 'at cost' was a major humanitarian legacy of COVAX and the Oxford-AZ vaccine. Yet it received little publicity. Perhaps British ministers were embarrassed by such public sector idealism.
- Unfortunately, there was also evidence of vaccine hoarding by wealthy nations. Some surplus vaccines 'donated' to developing countries had to be destroyed as they were beyond their 'sell-by' date.

Having got the vaccines, the NHS then delivered our vaccination programme with great success, largely due to its accurate computer database that provided contact details for all those prioritized for vaccines. (This contrasts with the earlier government-imposed NHS computer system that was aborted after wasting more than £4 billion).

Johnson, basking in the success of this vaccination programme, reportedly boasted to his MPs that success was due, not to public sector efficiency, but to capitalism and greed. Such self-delusion, almost childish in its naivety, slanders the real heroes.

The victims

If the UK government had been more competent with PPE and T&T, more flexible and more engaged with local expertise, then our Covid mortality rate would not have been among the highest in Europe. We should have done more to protect key frontline workers not just in hospitals and care homes, but also in buses, shops and schools etc. Apart from frontline workers, the following were most vulnerable to Covid infection.

In Europe, 90 per cent of those dying of Covid were over 60 years old; over half were 80 plus (Europe 2020). Put bluntly, nature has a way of 'thinning out' high-density populations, particularly of the old and infirm.

Pneumonia used to be called 'the old man's friend'. But today we can mitigate pandemics; failing to protect care home staff and residents was culpable.

We ignored early care home deaths; PPE and on-site testing were virtually non-existent, low-paid staff were expected to get to out-of-town drive-through testing sites until late summer, and residents were quarantined from loved ones in their last months of life, even when those visitors had tested Covid-free. This Spartan treatment was inhuman set against the many cheerful Downing Street parties – and incompetent. One *Private Eye* correspondent wrote that, while 125 deaths were recorded in 15 private care homes in Ealing, there were no infected residents in 17 council-run care homes in the Danish town where he lived, with their PPE and regular testing. This contrast between municipal and privatized public services is discussed further in Chapter 3.

Having stopped all visits to care homes, the government then ordered hospitals to release recovering Covid patients, often untested, into those care homes. This is denied by the government. Remarkably, the official inquiry, intent on gaining access to all relevant government information, may well uncover the truth in such matters. There is another question. Osborne's austerity having reduced hospital beds, why didn't the private hospitals offer their surplus beds?

Poverty increases vulnerability. About six million households, dependent on the simplified Universal Credit (UC), received a temporary £20 'uplift'. This only restored UC in line with inflation, but was then brutally withdrawn at the end of October 2121. Though the Chancellor later introduced a slight 'taper relief' for those actually working, there was no relief for those who can't work. Such meanness didn't stop there.

When UC was introduced, disabled people were left with their existing disability benefits. These had no uplift, despite disabled people being vulnerable to infection. Their benefits are also under continual review by private outsourcers, including Capita, Atos and Maximus. In five years, 5,600 disabled people have died within six weeks of their benefits and/or mobility allowances being reduced or stopped altogether, often with no medical professional present at the assessments.

The DWP (department for work and pensions) doesn't seem to know whether the deaths are related to the decisions, nor how many were suicides.

And, due to 'commercial confidentiality', we don't know whether the companies' annual multi-million pound dividends are a reward for reducing the 'tax burden' of those essential benefits, and/or simply the profit from employing low-paid unqualified staff. It is obscene when set beside about 1,000 mostly unjustified tax allowances for wealthy corporations and individuals – including a tax allowance for private chauffeurs. Taxing such 'expenses of wealth' might even restore mobility allowances for the disabled.

Low-paid workers were also vulnerable. In particular, ethnic minorities tend to be poorer pro-rata than the ethnic majority, and more likely to be exposed in low-paid frontline jobs in health, care and transport. Afro-Caribbeans experienced specific vulnerabilities:

- they seem to have lower immunity levels, which might have been alleviated during Covid with vitamin D tablets;
- they were more reluctant to be vaccinated (perhaps for historic reasons); and
- though hard evidence is scarce, these British citizens might simply be less resistant to infection living under the constant stress of covert discrimination, frequent outbreaks of naked racism and the government's own 'hostile environment'.

That 'hostile environment' from 2012, threatening to deport about 15,000 black UK citizens, was dubbed 'inhumane, inefficient and unlawful'. Most had been raised and taught here, before settling down to work, pay taxes and raise families. Sending them back to those countries where their parents or grandparents came from completes this racist circle of malevolence – many of them had been invited here by 'the right honourable' health minister Enoch Powell.

Many workers were exploited during Covid. To protect profits at the expense of wages, some profitable companies quietly fired and rehired staff on lower wages until P&O hit the headlines. In one government department, apparently, cleaners were expected to do their work in half the time – and half the pay. Can this be true? When the HGV driver shortage arose, the transport minister initially suggested increasing the daily shift from 9 to 10 hours. This put corporate interests before personal health and road safety, which might be thought a transport minister's primary concerns.

It gets worse. Workers having to isolate would receive their normal company sick pay. For low-paid staff in the gig economy or working with companies on government contracts like T&T, however, their pay was reduced to the statutory sick pay of £95 a week. And after a year of unparalleled staff shortages and sick leave, mental stress and physical exhaustion, nurses were offered a 1 per cent pay rise, later increased to 3 per cent. Leaving them significantly poorer after five years of inflation with no pay rise is social injustice.

Finally, the impact of Covid on three other groups is intangible. First were all those who 'lost' loved ones, particularly parents, spouses and even children, without being allowed to visit them in their last months of life.

Then many healthy young and middle-aged adults who were infected, suffered 'long Covid', with debilitating symptoms similar to ME, and as difficult to explain. Setting these patients on gentle physical exercise regimes helped some, but only made others worse.

It is impossible to gauge how children were affected. Few were infected, but a term not at nursery and reception deprives all pupils of their first experience of organized social life. Other 'rites of passage', moving to secondary school, taking exams and going to university, were seriously disrupted. Lockdowns affected them all, but for those living in poverty, free school meals were withdrawn until the footballer Marcus Rashford intervened – not once but twice. School holiday meals and vouchers illustrated the 'trickle-down' effect: the meagre portions of food for children contrasted with the greedy 'back siphonage' of profits on the public contracts.

For those learning to speak English, living in one-room 'temporary accommodation' or in abusive households, remote teaching at home for such long periods, particularly without laptops promised by the government, will affect their learning, mental health, social progress and future prospects in ways that are impossible to predict or evaluate when this form of 'long Covid' becomes apparent some years hence. Then, when they try to access underfunded child and mental health services, they will realize just how marginal they are in society.

As with care homes, the government did not protect schools from the real harm of lockdowns. Teachers, like bus drivers, shop staff and other key frontline workers were not prioritized for PPE and testing, and classrooms lacked adequate air ventilators to permit safe classroom activity. Eventually the government ordered 7,000 – for more than 300,000 classrooms in England. This could have been an opportunity for UK firms, though many were expensive Dyson ventilators imported from the far east.

In summary, Covid highlighted how underfunded the NHS and Social Services are to cure our ills and care for our old and infirm. And public health, in which prevention is both cheaper and more effective at improving personal health, is largely ignored. Consider each in turn.

The NHS

The NHS, one of our great political inventions, meets 'social demand'. Since 1979, however, it has been plagued by three serious problems: strategic underfunding, over-centralized management, and now privatization.

UK spending on health is lower than most of the 38 member states of the OECD. Per capita spending on health in 2006 was as follows (*The New York Times* (27/7/08):

- Spain $2,458, and Italy $2,614. The UK, not included, almost certainly spent less,
- Sweden, Denmark, Germany, Netherlands, France, Belgium, Austria and Canada ranged from $3,202 to $3,678,
- Switzerland $4,311, Norway $4,520, and the US $6,714 per head.

The *NY Times* commented that "… the United States spends much more on health care than other industrialized nations – … about twice the average in other countries – without providing better care". The EU *Health at a Glance: Europe 2020* confirms our chronic underfunding.

- In western Europe, Germany has 8 hospital beds/1,000 people, Austria 7.3, France 5.9, Belgium 5.6, Greece 4.2, Norway and Portugal 3.5, Netherlands 3.2, Italy 3.1, Spain and Ireland 3.0, Denmark 2.6, the UK 2.5, and Sweden 2.1. In other OECD nations, Japan has 13, South Korea 12.4 and the US 2.9 beds/1,000 (WHO).

- We also have fewer doctors than the rest of western Europe. Austria has 5.2/1,000 people, Portugal 5.2, Norway 4.8, Germany and Sweden 4.3, Denmark and Belgium 4.2, Italy and Spain 4.0, Netherlands 3.7, Ireland 3.3, France 3.2 and the UK 2.8. If our GPs had more than seven minutes to discuss each patient's problems, this might gradually improve our overall well-being and reduce the number of A&E admissions – if indeed prevention and cure are inversely correlated.
- The same is true for nurses. Our 7.3 nurses/1,000 compares with a European average of 8.2. High levels of staff vacancies affect all health sectors, compounded by Brexit when many European health workers returned home. Lest we forget, staff shortages rendered the ten Nightingale hospitals unusable.

As well as adequate funding, the government must ensure that the NHS is 'balanced'. Our mental health services are seriously underfunded, as they are throughout Europe, when compared, for example, with expensive cancer drug treatments that seldom add quality years to patients. Similarly, old people receive more generous treatment than the young. These are difficult issues.

Emergency services are chronically underfunded. With fewer staff and resources to deal with increasing demand, too many coroners' reports now include a 'prevention of future deaths report' which most hospital trusts are unable to address.

Despite inadequate resources and staff stressed beyond reasonable limits, governments persist with disruptive 'management reforms'. Under Thatcher, Keith Joseph imposed three tiers of bureaucracy. New Labour wasted at least £4 billion on a national computer system before it was abandoned, and introduced the inflated costs of all PFI (private finance initiative) contracts. Under the Coalition, Andrew Lansley set up 'internal markets… to drive efficiency and cut costs' under the *Health and Social Care Act 2012*. These privatized at least 7 per cent of the NHS budget, and rising. Under Cameron, Jeremy Hunt not only reduced hospital beds, but sought a fully functional seven-day-week hospital service, with no extra funds. And throughout, amateurs (aka management consultants) charged extortionate fees to show hospitals how to do more with even less money.

Incredibly, in the midst of the Covid crisis, the government imposed its own health reforms. PHE … was simply abolished. The back story on this reform must be published. Its replacement, the Health Security Agency, combines the PHE with the NHS T&T operation. The *Health and Care Act* 2022 now increases the health minister's control of the health service, and insists that private companies sit on all the new local Integrated Care Systems.

Covid simply provided an opportunity to privatize more health services. The new chair of NHS England, Richard Meddings, is a banker from Standard Chartered, TSB and now Credit Suisse [!] (*Private Eye* 1566). Meddings also advised Gordon Brown on strategy following the Bankers' Crash, which neither offered the banks commercial loans rather than capital 'bailouts', nor subsequently reformed them.

Two examples suggest poor value for money from private health providers. First, the government paid £2.15 billion to private hospitals (*Private Eye* 1561), including: £468.1 million to the US firm Circle Health Holdings Ltd, £430 million to the UK Spire Healthcare plc, and £385 million to the Australian-owned Ramsay Health Care UK Operations Ltd. Yet according to a report from the Centre for Health and the Public Interest, with their total of almost 8,000 beds, the private hospitals "provided only 3,000 of the 3.6 million Covid bed days in those 13 months – just 0.08% of the total." (*The Guardian* 7/10/21) This is extraordinary.

The report also stated that private hospitals carried out very few operations from the NHS backlog because NHS surgeons that private hospitals normally employ under contract were unavailable during Covid. We need to know what private hospitals did for their fees, how the services were monitored, and what 'claw-back' provisions were specified against non-delivery. If private hospitals delivered even less support than usual, wasting £2.15 billion would insult staff and taxpayers. Perhaps it's what the Brexit bus meant to say – £35 million a week to privatized NHS services.

Privatized GP surgeries confirm poor service. The large US health insurance Centene Corporation, acting as Operose Health, already 'owns' 70 GP surgeries (making it the biggest 'partner' with the NHS). During the first lockdown, it bought 37 London GP surgeries from AT Medics, a private company owned by six GPs. AT Medics had already extracted £35 million from the surgeries over the previous five years – nearly £190,000 each year from each surgery. "According to Allyson Pollock, clinical professor of public health at Newcastle University and author of the book *NHS plc*: "These deals are bad news for patients. The shareholders want a return on their investment. If the US experience is anything to go by, they pave the way for closure of surgeries, fewer GPs, lower staffing levels, reduced access to services, and erosion in quality of care and coverage"." (*Private Eye* 1543)

This was confirmed by a BBC *Panorama* programme (13/6/22) on Operose Health. Chronic lack of GPs, reliance on largely unsupervised 'physician assistants', huge backlogs of patients awaiting appointments, all to maximize profits and largely unregulated by the Care Quality Commission.

Inferior private GP services emerged well before Covid. "In Derbyshire the regional health authority put two village GP surgeries (in Creswell and Langwith) out to tender. This was won by an American healthcare company (UnitedHealth Europe) which beat, among others, a realistic bid from the local GPs with local support that included rebuilding the inadequate surgery in Langwith. A resident took the case to the High Court on the grounds of inadequate public involvement and won on appeal. When the contract was re-tendered,... the new tender was won by another healthcare company (ChilversMcCrea). According to their website "The key qualification for our team members is that we have all been round the block, are expert in what we do and are great fun to work with. There is no other team like it in the healthcare consultancy world."

"Needless to say, the Langwith surgery remained inadequate and the private company had difficulty finding qualified GPs in Creswell. Complaints rose, many locals de- registered and ChilversMcCrea sold the contract on to The Practice group, another private company. Whatever the problems, the private companies probably still made profits while the NHS could book some short-term savings in providing the GP services. Entirely lost to the two villages are the social and economic benefits of local health workers running their own GP services more effectively, supported by patients, parish councils and residents, plus a slightly stronger local economy." (*Civilizing Cities*)

Now, the purchase of those 37 London GP surgeries by Operose is also being challenged in the High Court. To anticipate Chapter 3, historic research from Michigan university found that public services under municipal control "... have, in addition to the purely business side (profit and loss)... a greater deal of attention paid to social aspects, such as better facilities to the consuming public and better compensation to the employees."

Failures in private health services are not widely reported. A Care Quality Commission report in 2018 found that two out of five private hospitals don't meet safety standards, there is little oversight of the 'independent' consultants, and when operations go wrong, the NHS has to take over. Putting profit before safety is hardly *efficient*.

The US private health system, consuming an extraordinary 18 per cent of national GDP, is grossly inefficient. With some of the best-equipped hospitals and doctors' surgeries in the world, its healthcare is riddled with unnecessary procedures and operations, excessive management costs, bureaucracy and fees, and largely ignores the poor. Prioritizing private wealth (through lower taxes) over universal access to an essential public service does not promote a healthy society.

The NHS, under rigorous cost controls, doesn't have the resources for unnecessary procedures – nor the ethical vacuum. In essence, private hospitals need to operate to make money, public hospitals need money to operate. This contrast between private sector profit focus and public service cost control is discussed further in Chapter 3.

Our care homes, for old people, the disabled and children at risk, are also seriously underfunded. Care staff are among the lowest-paid workers in the UK, and while many care homes are well-run, private equity homes pay out excessive unearned dividends, while being saddled with huge and ever-increasing debt burdens. While Tory governments usually solicit votes from the older half of society, here they promote libertarian values of low taxes over properly-funded care homes for the old and infirm.

Local public health

"Prevention is better than cure."

A new hospital offers politicians photo opportunities, even when it is only a new wing for which funding was approved many years previously. Public health is the Cinderella of the British health service, all-encompassing but vague. It includes "epidemiology, preventive medicine, planning the delivery of health care, communicable disease control, and environmental health." (*Penguin Encyclopedia*) Perhaps if we shift the emphasis from trauma to fitness, we would reduce hospital visits and make people happier.

A former colleague suggested that public health might best be understood as six overlapping tiers of personal, social and professional 'interventions'.

1. Self-help assumes personal responsibility for one's own health and fitness, through diet, exercise and other 'lifestyle' choices, based on information and understanding.
2. Social activities develop levels of social skills and friendships. They include community groups based on hobbies and sports, toddlers, youth clubs, self-help and local campaign groups. Councils offer swimming pools, youth services, adult education, libraries and public transport, while shops, pubs and work also develop public trust and 'social health'.
3. Regular health checks by GPs, chiropodists, dentists, district nurses and opticians, assess one's personal health. Also, government information and regulation to reduce smoking and gambling, etc.
4. A first tier of medical intervention is GP advice on specific personal health problems, including suitable activities from the previous tiers, a course of drugs, 'alternative therapies', or referral to specialist services.
5. Hospital treatment, whether through GP referral or direct to A&E, is for serious physical and mental disorders, with operations, intensive care and recovery beds.
6. Finally, long-term care is essential for children at risk, the disabled and all those who can no longer live independently.

The first four tiers roughly equate to preventive or primary healthcare. Ignore the first three, and problems stack up in the second three. Prevention is usually better than cure, and cheaper. Local GPs are the vital link between public health and intensive treatment, and public health strategies are probably best developed, and certainly best delivered, through local councils.

The only active role for government in public health is to regulate those industries that positively cause harm and increase hospital admissions. When health minister Hunt proposed his hospital 'reform', asking already overburdened staff to provide a seven-day service with no extra funding, staff or facilities, during the public consultation, I suggested that he should instead try to reduce hospital admissions by regulating key commercial interests. Taxing the junk food industry on its saturated use of fats, sugars, salt and advertising would help to reduce child obesity and hospital treatment of diabetics. He might also ask the transport minister to improve public transport to reduce road traffic, air pollution and consequent hospital admissions for patients with cardiovascular and respiratory failures. There was no reply.

Since 1979, governments resist regulating mega-corps that cause ill health, as evidenced by their tardy controls on smoking, gambling, strong alcohol, leaded petrol and adverts. This demonstrates the power of mega-corp marketing through 'hospitality', 'public relations', elite 'sponsorships' and 'political donations', or bribes in plain English (ipE).

Governments also ignore the potential for improving local public health, or forbid it.

- Before Thatcher was education minister, every pupil had free milk and every school meal had to provide half their daily nutritional needs. Since Thatcher, milk has gone, and meals declined to junk status with turkey twizzlers and fizzy drinks – increasing child obesity, hospital admissions and private profits.
- Vital ancillary education services need to be restored, including more teaching support staff, back-up professional services like tutors, school nurses and 'ed psychs', plus 'peripherals' like sport, music and residential centres.
- In transport, the only rational economic, environmental and social policy is to reduce road traffic and pollution, with better public transport and safe pedestrian and cycle networks (see Chapter 2).

- In economic development, we should replace inward global investment and the gig economy, and focus on internal growth with local firms enriching work by innovating and replacing imports (see Chapter 3).
- Public libraries, leisure centres and swimming pools (essential aspects of education in ancient Greece) must be rescued from near oblivion following the Bankers' Crash and Osborne's malicious austerity.
- Similarly, youth services, family centres and community development must be revived, not just to reduce street crime and anti-social behaviour and provide relevant support for those with serious personal problems, but also to develop the positive potential of young people and local communities.

All of the above relate to the *Marmot Review on Health Inequality* in Chapter 4.

Their relevance here is this. It is *only* in local councils that these disparate services can be effectively co-ordinated for maximum impact. Public health, including all those aspects mentioned earlier (and more), requires a 'collegiate' approach by teams of experts with local experience, all under local democratic control.

Within government health spending, there is considerable scope for devolution. In 2007/8, it spent £103.5 billion on the NHS (plus £1.2 billion on social care), while local councils spent £25.4 billion on social care services. In broad terms, this is an 80 per cent-20 per cent split between NHS and social services, or central and local government.

Back in 1976, my uncle John Pemberton (in *The Milroy Lecture* 1976; *Journal of the Royal College of Physicians*, Oct.1976) estimated that health spending in 1973/4 was broken down as follows:

- diagnosis and treatment 73 per cent, included hospitals (57 per cent), drugs (9 per cent) and general practice (7 per cent);
- prevention 6 per cent, included public health and health education (0.03 per cent); and
- social services 21 per cent, which included dentists and opticians.

This roughly confirms the 80/20 split between NHS and social services. My uncle thought a more effective distribution of funding would be hospitals 44 per cent, drugs 5 per cent, with GP, public health and health education each on 10 per cent, leaving social services on 21 per cent. That move towards prevention, however optimistic, clearly hasn't happened. It may have got worse.

It is inefficient for the government to control all health spending, leaving social services to underfunded local councils. All primary healthcare, from self-help and social activities to health checks and GP services, should be devolved to local authorities. Councils would ensure far better co-ordination between all public health services including GPs, cottage hospitals, care homes, community nursing, recreation, schools, education psychologists and youth services, and *chronic* medical treatment.

The sheer size of the NHS makes for mismanagement. Like the former British Rail, it needs splitting up into more focussed and manageable sectors. With perhaps 20 per cent of the NHS budget devolved to local councils to improve primary healthcare, responsibilities might be split as follows:

- the government would retain overall responsibility for health strategy and preventive medicine, university teaching hospitals, drug safety and audit functions;
- strategic cities and counties could manage and better integrate public health, trading standards and care homes with local hospitals; while
- most parish councils could manage their GP surgeries, as suggested earlier. Larger town councils might also manage care homes and cottage hospitals.

Local councils and GPs are crucial for all primary healthcare services, with many councils needing perhaps a five year transition period. But most of these services are precisely what they provided before World War II. While GP services were private and expensive, most councils ran isolation and cottage hospitals as well as health centres. With local democratic control over public health, smaller hospitals, social care and GPs, many of the major NHS scandals would have been reduced in scale, addressed more quickly, or even avoided altogether.

Welfare benefits, totalling £159.8 billion in 2007/8, might also benefit from devolution. If at least disability benefits, then more than £17 billion, were delegated through local councils with GPs and district nurses, etc., most would manage them more efficiently and humanely than the current private companies.

Devolving more health services would also ensure more innovation. The Finsbury public health centre, built in 1935 and managed by the council, was only one of many ground-breaking public health initiatives.

Today, many GPs are trying to reduce our dependence on drugs like antibiotics. A more recent initiative comes from a GP surgery in Southport. When a patient with type 2 diabetes complained to her doctor about the 'useless' medicine and had changed her diet, "Dr David Unwin... championed a low-carb lifestyle that not only helps patients lose weight [with weekly group sessions] but also, in more than half of his patients who were on the diet, has even managed to reverse type 2 diabetes, once thought to be an irreversible and progressive disease." (*The Observer,* 9/4/23) This treatment saves the surgery about £68,000 per annum on its drugs bill. Local councils might dovetail this success with more nutritious school meals, etc. Whether the government promotes this sustainable policy to reduce obesity and diabetes throughout Britain depends in part on its relations with the pharmaceutical mega-corps (see Chapter 3).

A long-term strategy to improve our health services should include the following:

- increase funding,
- devolve primary healthcare to local councils, leaving national strategy, drug regulation and teaching hospitals with the government, and
- gradually shift the emphasis from the cure of patients to improving public health.

What does public health mean? As distinct from genetic disorders and drug disasters (like Down's syndrome and Thalidomide) that are confined to individuals and their families, public health concerns those diseases that affect society at large. There are three categories of 'social disease'; infectious, contagious and psychosomatic.

- Infectious diseases like flu, measles and tuberculosis are spread by those already infected. Great strides have been made to control them, until a plague like Covid emerges that overwhelms societies.

- Contagious diseases are spread through external contamination rather than human contact. Polluted water spread cholera in mid-Victorian times, while today traffic pollution causes asthma and the premature death of thousands. The liberty of motorists reduces the social equity of residents, as discussed in the next chapter.
- Psychosomatic (lit mind/body) diseases have no clear bug or poison. It is how the mind reacts to any mix of social stress factors and how these might affect the body. Social factors include the social isolation of suburban life and car dependency, work that involves 'command management' and the gig economy is stressful rather than fulfilling (Chapter 3), while poverty causes parental stress and handicaps the mental and physical development of their children (Chapter 4). Perhaps worst are the advertisers who manipulate all our insecurities through peer pressure and pester power etc. Even children are exploited to eat junk food, drink alco-pops and gamble with their money and lives.

Whether such factors underlie strokes and cancers, or mental problems and suicide, etc., is of course vigorously contested. But like drugs, we need to curb or regulate the liberty of mega-corps to maximize profits at the risks of social and personal harm. The cynical defence, that people should be free to choose, doesn't mask unscrupulous greed.

CHAPTER 2

Living within the planet's environmental limits

Environmental health

Covid was a direct threat to human lives, affecting most families and neighbourhoods. It also overwhelmed all hospitals, except private ones. All plagues, however, are largely temporary. Vaccines, public health measures and even, perhaps, improved immunity will help societies to moderate their impact.

The remaining chapters deal with other more indirect threats to public health, like the gig economy and wealth inequality. But the most serious challenge to a sustainable future for all is global warming.

Humans, perhaps the most intelligent species on earth, can explain the impact of our behaviour on the planet by 'using sound science responsibly'. But, despite being a social species, we seem unable to defuse the climate crisis and undo the damage. At the COP26 conference that the UK chaired in Glasgow in November 2021, it was 'one minute to midnight' in terms of urgency. Big words from little men, empty rhetoric for society.

If Covid arose out of our mistreatment of our environment, the climate crisis is an existential threat to the whole planet. Despite climate deniers (whose personal freedoms or corporate profits are threatened), rising temperatures, melting ice caps and frequent 'extreme weather events' confirm the global threat.

There is also a direct link between climate and health. In *The Milroy Lecture* quoted above, my uncle preferred Pavlov's (1928) definition of health – as "being in equilibrium with surrounding nature". Covid, in transferring disease from 'lower' animals to humans, merely illustrates just how unstable our relationship with nature has become. Plagues, 'zoonosis', are but one symptom of our relentless poisoning of air, land and water infecting all food chains, destroying natural habitats and biodiversity with the genocidal extinction of species – all accelerating global warming.

We are fouling our own nest. To Gaia, if she exists, we are the plague.

From the latest report of the IPCC (the International Panel on Climate Change, set up by the United Nations in 1988) "… we have to act, we need a whole of society approach, no one can be left out, no household, no businesses, no government…" The EU health guide clarifies the challenge. Covid "provides a unique opportunity to promote a green economic recovery by integrating environmental considerations in decision-making processes… and achieving the 2030 EU national emission targets."

Unfortunately, the UK government, having 'taken back control' following Brexit, has often brazenly fuelled the crisis and increased emissions.

All areas of public policy have some impact on 'the planet's environmental limits'. *Civilizing Cities* explores how suburban sprawl, slum clearance, foodsheds, globalization and transport all fuel global warming, but transport is the most critical. Actual CO_2 emissions in 2019 (365.1 $MtCO_2$) were distributed as follows: transport 33.0 per cent, energy supply 24.5 per cent, residential 18.2 per cent, business 17.8 per cent, public 2.2 per cent and other 4.1 per cent (Government Department of Business, Energy and Industrial Strategy). These figures vary slightly from year to year, but transport and energy supply account for well over half of our emissions. And these exclude all international flights to and from the UK – hardly 'using sound science responsibly'.

The following text, on private traffic, public transport, personal mobility and household emissions, illustrates two fundamental themes:

- the UK transport system prioritizes private traffic over all other modes of transport, in marked contrast to all other west European nations, and
- our reliance on 'market demand' is unsustainable in its profligate use of energy.

Private traffic

All cities developed as compact settlements of buildings providing shelter and private security, with roads providing access and social space. When the wheel, cart and horse combined, traffic congestion emerged – and highway planning.

- In mid-16th-century Rome, three new broad avenues linked the heart of the city and St Peters with the northern gateway, the Piazza del Popolo, relieving congestion from both foot pilgrims and wealthy residents' new horse-drawn carriages.
- Three centuries later, Baron Haussmann transformed Paris with a comprehensive web of boulevards. Discounting any military purpose, the city now had wide, tree-lined avenues to relieve traffic congestion, with a healthy network of sewers beneath. Urban life was largely confined to the areas within the boulevards.

In 20th-century Britain, two factors greatly increased road traffic; suburban sprawl and the motor car. In England and Wales, from 1901 to 2001, the population grew by 62 per cent (from 32,528,000 to 52,360,000) – a lower percentage increase than most west European nations. Yet our urban areas expanded roughly sixfold, to cover about 14,000 sq. km (9 per cent) of the total land area of 150,280 sq. km. By contrast, the Dutch population nearly trebled, while retaining compact cities with social neighbourhoods and pedestrian convenience.

Our desire for suburban privacy, inextricably linked with the comfort and status of cars, created an unhealthy 'positive feedback loop'. At low densities, buses pick up fewer passengers/mile, fares or subsidies rise, more passengers buy cars, buses lose more fares, services are reduced and 'car dependency' ensues. Suburbs lack the pedestrian convenience of local shops, businesses and social facilities, and waste precious land. This is unsustainable.

In 1963, Buchanan defined UK highway strategy in the *Traffic in Towns* report. It showed how to accommodate cars, "at no cost to the motorist", "with a radically new urban form". A century after Haussmann, his schemes for Newbury, Norwich, Leeds and a central London neighbourhood still shock those with a nervous disposition.

What gave Buchanan's report a professional gloss was its clear planning process: predict likely growth in car ownership and trip generation (between existing and likely new housing, shops and workplaces), and then provide the roads required. 'Predict and provide' planning simply reinforces 'market forces' based on questionable assumptions. Do we all want a car? Motorists should not be "obliged to pay the full economic costs of running their vehicles, including the rental of road space." Public transport was airily dismissed as lacking in comfort and convenience. Only one of the four schemes was costed with a dubious cost/benefit analysis, and the external costs were ignored, like replacing beneficial horse emissions with toxic car fumes. This also is unsustainable.

It is also inherently fascist to redesign cities solely for the convenience of motorists. However libertarian in spirit, the 'market demand' for these new 'freeways' relied on compulsory purchase powers to destroy too many buildings and neighbourhoods simply to provide ever-more road space and car parks.

60 years later, Covid gave us a rare and wonderful glimpse of what traffic reduction means. The dramatic reduction in cars and planes during the first lockdown, plus the silent building sites and parks, transformed our lives, albeit temporarily. We could now hear just how noisy the birds were, even though they were singing more quietly. As with light pollution, noise is a symptom of our disequilibrium with nature. Perhaps we should tax all energy use other than human muscle.

Low traffic didn't last and its positive impact was ignored by government. Today, road traffic has largely 'recovered' to former levels, unlike public transport, despite many people still working from home.

Table 2. Covid traffic in Great Britain as percentage of pre-Covid levels

	Cars	Vans	HGVs	All road	Rail	Buses	Cycles
6/4/20	34	42	61	37	5	11	105
6//7/20	79	93	97	83	19	29	138
5/10/20	86	103	106	91	34	33	95
11/1/21	56	79	97	63	14	26	70
6/4/21	75	95	98	80	24	36	58
5/7/21	93	110	108	98	49	60	88
11/10/21	94	111	110	98	69	80	83
10/1/22	82	103	102	87	56	68	86

Source: Department for Transport

(London Transport's tube and bus figures are similar to the national rail and bus figures.)

Table 3. Passenger transport in Great Britain, 1979–2019

Billion passenger km	1979 (% of total)	2019 (%)	2019 as % of 1979
Air (domestic only)	3 (0.6)	9 (1.0)	300%
Rail	35 (7.4)	80 (9.2)	229%
Road:			
• buses and coaches	56 (11.9)	33 (3.8)	59%
• cars, vans and taxis	365 (77.5)	738 (84.7)	202%
• motor cycles	7 (1.5)	5 (0.6)	71%
• pedal cycles	5 (1.1)	6 (0.7)	120%
All modes	471 (100)	871 (100)	185%

Source: Department for Transport

While private road transport is largely back to pre-Covid levels, buses have regained less than 75 per cent, trains less than 55 per cent of their former passengers. This trend was reinforced during lockdowns. UK government advice was to walk or cycle wherever possible, and avoid public transport, ignoring the safety of masks. Unlike the birds, it was silent on cars and planes. This reflects the ideological preference for private over public transport since 1963 and the power of the road and aviation lobbies.

Cars dominate British transport. Table 3 shows their 'market share' growing over 40 years by 7.2 percentage points, more than any other mode.

Comparative travel costs heavily favour motoring. Against a retail price index of 100 in 1987, the total costs of motoring (including purchase and maintenance, petrol, oil, tax and insurance) fell in 2017 to 90.3 per cent of their 1987 cost. During the same 30 years, rail fares rose by 145.5 per cent, bus and coach fares by 170.5 per cent (House of Commons Library: *Railways: fares statistics*).

From 1979 to 2019, annual road deaths reduced from almost 6,000 to well under 2,000. This major achievement conceals an uncomfortable truth. During that period, the total road network only increased by nearly 16 per cent (from 344,000 to 398,000 km, largely of minor roads), but licenced cars and vans more than doubled (16.8 to 36.0 million). More road congestion reduces average speeds and hence the severity of road crashes.

The corollary, unfortunately, is that more congestion increases pollution. "Across Europe, [there were] between 168,000 and 346,000 premature deaths due to air pollution from fine particulates alone in 2018." (*Health at a Glance: Europe* 2020) According to Treasury estimates, British road pollution kills about 40,000 people prematurely, second only to cancers and cardiovascular diseases. (British squirrels also suffer worse lung damage the closer they live to city centres.)

When the link between contaminated water supplies and cholera outbreaks was realized, Victorian councils quickly installed clean water supplies and sewers. For over 50 years, we have done nothing about traffic deaths. Perhaps we should 'bring back Victorian values'.

However approximate these death counts, we regularly exceed EU and WHO air quality standards. With Brexit, will we ignore them? The UK 'strategy' relies on electric cars (EVs) to improve air quality. This ignores serious problems.

- 36 million EVs averaging 10,000 miles per annum will put the national grid under severe strain, transferring most CO_2 emissions from cars to power stations.
- Many of the poisonous particulates come from brakes and tyres.
- Battery technologies rely on 'critical raw materials', rare metals of which China and the Democratic Republic of the Congo are major sources. The mining of these metals, like Nickel, will inevitably destabilize our links with the environment, destroying natural habitats, including rainforests, thereby increasing global warming and threatening native human settlements.

All cars have excessive embedded energy and their weight-to-load ratios are unsustainable compared with public transport, and off-the-scale when compared with bikes and shoes. EVs are even heavier and more inefficient. Cars also destroy residential streets as social space, drivers put on weight and car parks waste valuable land.

Driving is profoundly anti-social, displacing religion as 'the opium of the people'. Not all motorists are addicts. Most women regard their car as a tool, drive more slowly, and are thus safer drivers than men. For too many males, however, speed is their high. Look at their adverts. Unlike amphetamine addicts spurred into activity, drivers are more like Pavlov's dogs, swaddled in their bucket-seat wombs in air-conditioned exoskeletons, the adrenalin rush at the touch of the accelerator and, rather than a bell, the sound of the wind whistling past. Until he meets an impediment and throws a tantrum – like a low traffic neighbourhood (LTN) that some councils imposed during lockdown by closing residential streets to through-traffic, to prevent 'rat running'.

One August afternoon in 2020, during the first lockdown, we were drinking with friends in their front garden on the day that our council had closed four such rat runs that avoided a congested junction on the A2 south of our local park, and the congested town centre to the north. We were genuinely shocked at the anger of motorists when confronted with planters preventing their turning right into the residential street opposite our friends' home. Some swore loudly, most drove off recklessly, and two drivers actually got out, up-ended a planter and drove through. Within two minutes, four residents emerged to right the planter, earning loud abuse from new motorists and my congratulations on their polite responses. Are such motorists fit to drive?

With the side roads closed, the main street and its shops, cafes, pubs and primary school became much more sociable. With negligible traffic, we could walk in the middle of the side streets just like a century ago, while a few even jogged down the main street. All we needed now was to get rid of the parked cars!

Inevitably, a petition was organized to scrap the scheme, despite all residential streets west of the park now enjoying much less traffic intrusion, not just the four closed streets. Apparently, 28,000 extra vehicles were causing considerable congestion and delays on the two main east-west routes. In normal times, this congestion would ease back to previous levels. With government warnings to avoid public transport, however, and with extortionate train fares, few motorists are willing to leave their cars at home. But 28,000 vehicles is the capacity of a busy motorway lane. Surely no one believes that such traffic is acceptable in local streets. The council withdrew the scheme, promising to look at alternatives.

The real challenge, largely ignored, is how to reduce *all* road traffic. A common objection to road closures and LTNs is that emergency vehicles are delayed. This is true, but is tiny when compared with the delays to *all* emergency vehicles by general road congestion. Ambulances and fire engines used to be sent from two or three stations to keep response times below the 8-minute target, before Osborne's austerity closed down 'surplus' stations and reduced staff to provide basic skeleton services – and dangerously increased response times. Unnecessary road trips seriously disrupt emergency services most days, increasing risks to health and home in all urban areas.

The only serious policy to reduce traffic was in 1993, when John Major imposed an annual fuel duty 'escalator' to curb needless car trips. Abandoned in 2008, Sunak (in his first Covid budget) proudly refused to revive the escalator for five years and then, in 2022, reduced the tax by five pence a litre. With unparalleled government spending, this annual gift of perhaps £12 billion (and rising) mocks taxpayers and non-motorists, and ingratiates Sunak with his wealthy chums in their 'gas guzzling' four-wheel drive 'Chelsea tractors'.

In that budget, he also allocated £27 billion for major new roads. £10 billion of this was reshuffled from other budgets but, incredibly, another £5.5 billion was from carbon reduction measures. From Buchanan's love of cars, UK governments now fear motorists and the roads lobby. They even promote new roads as job creation schemes, which in truth are only a few low-skilled jobs. Investing £27 billion in upgrading railways and renovating vacant homes would increase skilled jobs and wages, provide useful outputs, and strengthen local economies rather than corporate profits.

There is another problem. To approve a major road scheme, the 'virtual time savings' must exceed the road's 'design cost'. Once approved, invariably the actual cost rises substantially, making a mockery of the cost/benefit analysis and approval. If this government's proposed roads are approved, my estimate of 'cost creep' (and corporate greed) will raise final costs from £27 billion to over £45 billion.

Reversing this 'virtual time saving' analysis, we could estimate a 'virtual time cost' of motoring. For example, about 12 million UK commuters drive to work. If their two daily trips average 1.5 hours over 250 workdays, the total drive time is 4.5 billion hours. At a less than average salary of £20/hour, the annual cost of commuting by car exceeds £90 billion. That could justify a substantial investment in buses and trains, walking and cycling.

New roads can no longer be justified by 'virtual' time savings over existing roads. All drive time is 'dead time', being unproductive, polluting, dangerous and unsustainable. It contradicts the *Climate Change Act* 2008 and fuels the climate crisis.

Before discussing better public transport and safe bike and pedestrian networks to curb automania, nowhere is UK government contempt for the climate crisis clearer than in its **aviation policy**. Though technically aviation is public transport, it is subject to the same 'predict and provide' strategy as private road traffic.

We must update our estimates of aviation emissions. For decades, plane contrails of water vapour and soot particles have had an even greater impact on global warming than its carbon emissions. We must also include international flights in our national emissions.

From Table 3, domestic passenger flights have trebled since 1979. This is largely due to ever-increasing rail fares. Early this century, industry adverts in main rail stations boasted that over 80 per cent of inter-city trips are cheaper by air. Today, they're probably all much cheaper.

With Covid came a dramatic fall in flying and predictions of a slow market recovery to pre-Covid levels. Those of us under busy flight paths could now enjoy time out in gardens, allotments, parks and streets without the intrusive roar of aircraft. Here was a real opportunity to reset aviation policy. Raising or increasing taxes on frequent flyers, domestic flights, private jets, night flights, first class travel or even just on kerosene would have sent a clear message. Real taxes would reduce flights and encourage rail trips, video conferencing and local holidays.

While France reduced domestic flights, Chancellor Sunak actually reduced their taxes in his November 2021 budget. This makes fiscal sense, since civil servants take about 250,000 domestic flights a year. Rather than go by train, they prefer to fly in the face of the climate crisis. Sustainable?

The UK government is afraid to produce its airport strategy. "In early 2020, every significant commercial airport in the UK had expansion plans." (*Private Eye* 1567) All were put on hold, but no longer. Leeds Bradford, Liverpool John Lennon, London City, Luton and Marston airports have all revived their plans, and expansion plans for Bristol and Southampton airports have been approved. While the Southampton decision is facing legal challenge, at Bristol, the planning inspectors stated that, without government policy on aviation, legal targets to reduce CO_2 emissions must be met elsewhere.

This illustrates a cynical twist to central government power: because it can't produce a sustainable airport strategy, planning inspectors can't follow the science either. (This silence on key environmental policies is rich, alongside perpetual government harassment of local councils to produce local plans and keep them up-to-date.) This may explain the eerie silence on the proposed third Heathrow runway, despite the High Court dismissing it on environmental grounds. (Johnson now supports the runway, following a deal that, before every first class flight from Heathrow, he enjoys – free – a £1,800 'Windsor Suite' service for VIPs involving expensive food, personal butler, shopper and chauffeur to plane!)

Johnson and now Sunak believe in having cake and eating it. But while stuffing themselves, they are also pissing on everyone whose towns are occasionally flooded, whose forests are ablaze, whose farms are now deserts or under seawater, and whose homes are tossed in the air by tornadoes. (I did think that Johnson's verb 'spaff' would be less vulgar – until I looked it up!)

Public transport

If private transport is essentially libertarian, public transport by its very nature is social, whether by train or metro, bus or tram.

Traffic in Towns sought to make cities accessible to all road traffic, at no cost to motorists. *The Reshaping of British Railways* (also in 1963, and chaired by ICI director Dr Beeching) sought to make the railways profitable – by removing a third of the network. This early example of government confidence in commercial acumen rather than professional expertise, was also a glaring conflict of interest. Both reports were commissioned by the Minister of Transport, Ernest Marples, from the major road contractor Marples-Ridgeway. Road traffic was paramount, whatever the cost. National railways are only profitable when 'full cost accounting' is used.

Compared with the 'dead time' of road trips, rail trips are safe, quick, less polluting, more productive and sustainable. Improving rail services and reducing fares would reduce long-distance road traffic and the 'demand' for new roads. Despite Beeching, from 1976, the InterCity 125 high-speed trains were an almost instant success and imitated throughout Europe. They reinforced the integrity of the whole network, with central stations retained as major interchanges for local trains as well as social locations with bars and cafes for relaxed meetings and greetings. And when British Rail (BR) was split into four operational divisions – InterCity, Southeast, Cross Country and Rail Freight – it became much more efficient, reducing subsidies to about 20 per cent of operating costs, and confirming the efficiency of smaller, more focussed businesses discussed in the next chapter.

BR used to be quasi-independent of government except for subsidy support and infrastructure investment, its professional expertise comparable to that of the BBC. That efficiency was lost when it was privatized by John Major in

1994. The trains were split into 14 franchises run by coach firms and European national rail companies, all leasing trains from three profiteering train leasing companies, and using the private rail and station infrastructure owned by Railtrack, until it went bust. Effectively, national rail is now a fully nationalized entity, managed by DfT (Department for Transport) civil servants with their legion of consultants and lawyers. Only rail expertise is missing – except in its own 'Railway Company' that runs failing rail franchises with greater efficiency and passenger satisfaction, until the government establishes a new franchise.

Table 4. European rail passenger traffic, 1900–2003

Nation	Passenger trips (millions)			Passenger km (billions) / av trip km 2003
	1900	1950	2003	
Austria	78.7	115.2	188	8.3 / 44
Belgium	139.1	219.1	152.5	8.0 / 53
Denmark	20.8	111.0	162.6	5.5 / 34
Finland	7.1	46.3	59.8	3.3 / 56
France	430.0	545.0	906.0	73.5 / 81
Germany	856.0	2,426	1,600	70.7 / 44
Greece	6.2	–	8.7	1.5 / 172
Ireland	27.7	11.4	34.6	1.6 / 46
Italy	59.7	527.1	504.3	45.6 / 90
N'lands	30.8	158.4	320.0	14.3 / 45
Norway	7.0	40.1	38.6	2.4 / 63
Portugal	11.9	57.5	160.1	3.9 / 25
Spain	32.0	107.5	401.2	19.3 / 48
Sweden	30.8	150.0	148	9.1 / 61
Switzerland	62.2	267.6	327	14.5 / 44
UK	1,114.6	704.0	1,012	40.9 / 40

Source: Mitchell; European Historical Statistics

Comparing west European railways shows that, over the last century, passenger growth occurred in all nations except the UK: 10 per cent growth in Belgium, 20 per cent in Greece and Ireland, double in France and Germany, fivefold in Denmark, Finland, Italy, Norway, Sweden and Switzerland, and more than tenfold in the Netherlands, Portugal and Spain.

Unlike Europe, UK passenger numbers have only returned to the heyday of the 1920s – hardly the success that some claim. To put it in perspective, the London Underground carries as many passengers. When Major promised that within five years, the railways would be subsidy-free, operating subsidies ballooned from about 20 per cent under BR, to nearer 50 per cent. These figures are mired in controversy, however, abetted by commercial confidentiality and creative accounting. Even passenger numbers may be inflated, for example by multiple tickets for single and return trips involving more than one train company. BR statistics were trustworthy.

What is clear is that passenger fare income almost trebled at 2017/8 prices between 1987 and 2017 – from £3,311 million to £9,655 million. Since 2002, subsidies have exceeded £5 billion per annum, reaching £8 billion in 2006/7 and £7.1 billion in 2018/9 (*Wikipedia*). Much of this subsidy has been invested in costly infrastructure upgrades, all undertaken by private companies with few skills but rampant cost creep, inflated management fees, excessive subcontracting and cost overruns. BR would have invested such generous subsidies much more efficiently, using its in-house workforce of skilled engineers, buying new trains rather than leasing them, replacing diesel trains with cleaner more efficient electric trains, and reinvesting profits from popular routes rather than paying out dividends. It would have managed the suppressed demand better, with much cheaper and more rational fares, and less overcrowding of trains, without compromising safety or fragmenting services.

Perversely, even during Covid when the railways were struggling to attract passengers back onto trains, the annual fare escalator above the RPI (retail prices index) was maintained – even as the motorists' fuel tax escalator was dropped. Government support for public transport operators was also partial. In March of the first lockdown, the rail franchisees were given prompt financial support, making them greater profits during Covid than before, despite their dramatic loss of passengers. Yet apparently, the local Merseyrail franchise, controlled by the Merseyside PTE (passenger transport executive), while outperforming all other rail franchisees with the best punctuality, lowest fares/mile and highest passenger satisfaction ratings, had to wait until May for any support, alongside city transport networks. Transport for London was refused any support until it agreed to increase all its fares. Such malice undermines local democracy.

UK rail freight is similarly blighted.

Table 5. European rail freight traffic ('000 tonnes), 1900–2003

Nation	1900	1950	2003 (million tonne km)
Austria	25.3	35.9	91.3 (17.6)
Belgium	55.1	60.0	60.5 (7.1)
Denmark	4.2	9.3	7.9 (1.9)
Finland	2.5	16.8	42.7 (10.1)
France	83.4	152.0	142 (50.0)
Germany	360.3	419.5	384 (78.5)
Greece	0.3	1.9	0.4 (0.5)
Ireland	5.2	3.6	2.1 (0.4)
Italy	18.0	50.5	83.1 (23.3)
N'lands	18.0	50.5	83.1 (23.3)
Norway	1.6	14.6	19.4 (2.6)
Portugal	2.7	3.3	10.7 (2.5)
Spain	31.5	29.8	32.9 (11.9)
Sweden	21.6	44.1	60 (20.9)
Switzerland	14.5	24.0	62.4 (10.6)
UK	426.5	285.8	142 (18.7)

Source: Mitchell; European Historical Statistics

Continental Europe enjoys an integrated rail network and increased total rail freight tonnage by 63 per cent over the last century. In smaller nations, most rail freight is in transit between their larger neighbours which enables Switzerland, for example, to impose severe restrictions on road haulage and HGVs.

By contrast, rail freight tonnage in Ireland and the UK declined dramatically. The irony is that, in their early years, British Rail companies refused to carry passengers (until forced to by law) because they interfered with the profitable freight business. Since 1979, rail freight has been wilfully neglected, or subjected to 'market forces':

- Daily newspapers used to be distributed on the night mail trains, until Murdoch did a deal with an Australian road haulier;
- Red Star used to deliver parcels by train. You could even hand in a parcel at your station, for it to be collected by the addressee at their nearest station;
- In 1982, there were 339 rail freight depots and marshalling yards for heavy bulk goods. In 1993, there were just 61 (ONS);
- For example, Smithfield market used to have its own basement rail link for beef and lamb from the whole of Britain. Now it is a disco. All meat arrives in 40-tonne refrigerated HGVs in the early morning; and
- Rail freight charges, although paying less than the full costs of wear and tear on the tracks, are still paying far higher access charges than 40 tonne HGVs that impose far higher costs on society in terms of congestion, road damage, crashes and pollution.

Higher freight charges by both road and rail would actually benefit local businesses by reducing the profits of foodsheds and those national firms that buy out local bakers and brewers, etc., closing local production with national distribution that stifles local competition.

Finally, the UK government persists with the ludicrous HS2 project, which was initially costed at £34.5 billion. Its cost has crept in such leaps and bounds that it is likely to exceed £150 billion. HS2 will struggle to repay the interest charges let alone the capital costs. Nor will they reduce domestic flights without substantial fare reductions, making a double mockery of the 'cost-benefit analysis'.

High-speed rail services must be integrated with the existing network. In Burgos, Spain, having closed the central station and converted the railway into a local road, the new station, three miles out of town, attracts fewer passengers. In France, few new stations connect with central stations, so the regional and local networks attract fewer passengers.

Since 1970, the French rail network has shrunk from 36,530 km to 29,901 km in 2008 (International Union of Railways).

If HS2 were scrapped altogether, even at this late stage, the £100 billion + saved (plus the £27 billion from not building new roads) would electrify most or all of the network and reduce carbon emissions, relieve existing 'bottlenecks' and upgrade regional railways outside the southeast.

There is one positive feature with HS2. Its 'cost-benefit analysis' included not only time savings over existing rail services but also, for the first time, the real benefit of business passengers working on HS2. To be consistent, the government must now extend this benefit to all inter-city rail services where real working hours on the trains far outweigh the 'virtual' time savings (projected over 15 years, rather than 15 months or even less before congestion re-emerges to cancel those time savings) that dishonestly justify all new road schemes.

When Thatcher deregulated all bus services outside London in 1985, bus trips fell from 12 per cent to 4 per cent of all trips (Table 3). That conceals the discrepancy between professionally managed public bus services and profiteering private bus companies.

Table 6. British bus services and passenger trips, 1985/6–2008/9

Regions	1985/6	1992/3	2008/9
Local bus services (vehicle km millions)	2,077	2,515	na
London	273	330	
Metropolitan areas	574	678	
Shire counties	849	1,042	
Scotland	285	346	
Wales	95	118	
Local bus passenger trips (millions)	5,641	4,483	5,233
London	1,152	1,128	2,149
Metropolitan areas	2,068	1,386	1,111
Shire counties	1,588	1,308	1,355
Scotland	671	532	515
Wales	163	129	124
Passenger receipts (£mn)	2,219	3,033	na

Source: ONS, Annual Abstract

While London buses carry 86 per cent more passengers with more services and cheaper fares, elsewhere private bus companies have been hoovering profits while haemorrhaging passengers by 31 per cent. Ominously, statistics for total bus service kilometres and passenger fares are not available. While profits confirm the dogma of privatization, 'commercial confidentiality' conceals key information about staff pay, bus maintenance, pricing strategy and profit distribution. What is clear is that, outside the capital, maximizing fares and profits hit the poor hardest and increase car trips and road congestion.

In fact, cheaper fares could be more profitable. Prior to deregulation, municipal bus companies ran more buses on more routes with better paid drivers, lower fares and far more passengers. One major feature was that, instead of extracting up to 20 per cent of turnover as dividends, public bus companies re-invested all profits to upgrade the fleet and cross-subsidize some loss-making routes.

Buses highlight the contrast between libertarian dogma and social efficiency.

And finally, by about 1960, Britain had ripped out all of its tram and trolleybus systems to relieve congestion and free up roads for cars. Towns and cities now relied on buses and local trains, unlike the rest of Europe. For example, in Germany, 18 of its 19 largest cities have retained their extensive tram networks. Today, following their British 'renaissance', many miles of our meagre tram networks in Croydon, Manchester, Nottingham, Sheffield, the West Midlands and Edinburgh actually use existing railway lines. Trams should only run on roads, to reduce road traffic and relieve (not congest) the railways. To avoid the 'cost creep' of installing heavy trams, we might also restore the quieter, more flexible and even more energy-efficient trolleybuses.

Pedals and pedestrians

The UK government prioritizes private traffic over public transport, and largely ignores personal mobility on bike or foot – except when riding a bike presents a photo-opportunity. Yet walking and cycling are the most sustainable form of transport.

During Covid, it did encourage walking and cycling, but with some hypocrisy.

- In the first lockdown, we were urged to restrict our shopping to one trip a week. This describes a car trip to a foodshed. It is neither possible nor desirable for the rest of us who use local shops and markets to carry home a week's shopping in one trip.
- We were also forbidden to walk and socialize in parks.
- Yet, while walking and cycling are healthy, non-polluting and sociable, they are both dangerous. The government steadfastly refuses to promote and fund LTNs and safe walking and cycling networks, in fear of the road lobby.

In the first lockdown, bikes blossomed with the birdsong. From Table 2, during May 2020, weekday cycling was up on average by 177.5 per cent (and by 206 per cent in the final week of May). At weekends and bank holidays, it was often three times normal levels, averaging 273 per cent. This potential was ignored. By October 2020, cycling had slipped back into negative figures, averaging 80–85 per cent of former levels. This confirms just how threatening motorists are when cocooned in their exoskeletons, and HGVs.

Before 1900, our towns and cities were compact for pedestrian convenience. With suburban sprawl and traffic, however, cyclists and walkers became second class citizens, despite using the healthiest and most efficient transport modes. On all highways, we are regarded solely as a 'safety issue' rather than a legitimate highway user with equal rights of access.

- At most traffic signal-controlled junctions, cars have priority. Pedestrians are often diverted off their pavement route and even held in central reservations, having to wait for two 'green men'. Even in Trafalgar Square, cars and buses are given 75 seconds, while far more pedestrians then have 15 seconds.
- In Japan, apparently, most crossroads have four pedestrian crossings connecting the four pavements without deviation.
- In the Netherlands, cyclists have the right of way. In the event of a crash between car and bike, the motorist is held responsible. That encourages, or enforces, low traffic speeds. In the UK, until recently, councils were not allowed to impose 20 mph speed limits without government permission.

A general 20 mph speed limit in all urban areas, with 10 or 5 mph limits in residential streets, would not seriously affect average urban traffic speeds of 10–12 mph. British cities need safe pedestrian and cyclist networks, by converting perhaps a fifth of all urban streets and country lanes to pedestrian-priority networks. We also lack car-free residential areas, as in Germany and the Netherlands, even though in our towns and cities, up to 40 per cent of households have no car.

Integrating transport strategy

"Politics is not the art of the possible. It consists in choosing between the disastrous and the unpalatable." (JK Galbraith)

Our transport strategy is both. UK governments are afraid to address the libertarian 'market demand' for private traffic. Granting motorists free access to an ever-expanding road network, while raising fares in a vain attempt to make public transport 'subsidy-free', and ignoring the potential of bikes and pavements, is disastrous. Yet imposing fair taxes on road traffic to encourage public transport, walking and cycling is unpalatable. This is unsustainable.

It is also irrational. Most transport spending is on national roads and HS2. In 2007/8, it spent about £20 billion on transport, leaving £6.7 billion for local councils, roughly a 75 per cent-25 per cent split. Yet 75 per cent of all trips are less than five miles, and 25 per cent under one mile. As with health, it would be more rational to devolve more responsibility to subregional PTEs (passenger transport executives) and local councils. Consider the potential.

At the national level, the government would control the motorway and trunk road network, domestic flights and national rail services. To reduce road traffic, the government must restore the fuel tax escalator to former levels (but in a 'tax neutral' way, as discussed in Chapter 5), and encourage all councils to calm traffic. To reduce road freight, it must increase the annual HGV road tax to be significantly higher, not less, than rail access charges. It must also revive the professionalism of BR at least for InterCity, Cross Country and Rail Freight services.

These rail services would be more profitable if cars, HGVs and planes were taxed at least fairly to encourage more sustainable long-distance trips. Reducing motorway speeds (and hence the 'virtual time savings' of each trip) would also reduce emissions and encourage more trips by rail.

At the subregional level, like Merseyside and East Anglia, PTEs or local council partnerships could manage their regional rail networks, paying access charges to BR for the infrastructure of track and signals, trains and stations. And as many regional rail passengers 'feed' into InterCity services,

Living within the planet's environmental limits

so the profits of the latter might subsidize the former. PTEs could also provide more road and rail 'transhipment' depots to transfer far more HGV goods onto freight trains, with LGVs for local delivery.

Towns and cities would improve their urban transport systems and develop safe networks for cycling and walking. Table 7, compiling urban transport data for all west European cities with over 250,000 residents, shows the potential of public transport.

Table 7. Annual social transport urban trips by nation, 1983–2008

Nation	Total city populations	Total trips (millions) 1983	Total trips (millions) 2008	Percentage increase	2008, average trips/person
Austria	1.97	623.7	898.5	44.1	456.1
Belgium	1.472	251.0	456.5	81.9	310.1
Finland	0.565	168.4	188.1	11.7	332.9
France	2.224	521.1	840.7	61.0	378.0
Germany E	4.496	1,821.9	1,371.7	(-24.7)	305.1
Germany W	10.949	2,196.4	2,840.2	29.3	259.4
Greece	0.745	500	645.2	29.0	866.0
Ireland	0.506	159	148	(-6.9)	292.5
Italy	3.092	1,289.9	1,077.8	(-16.4)	348.6
Netherlands	2.26	421.7	469.7	11.4	207.8
Spain	3.485	642.2	984.0	53.2	282.4
UK	2.556	730.8	536.3	(-26.6)	209.9

Based on data sourced in Jane's Urban Transport Systems

(Urban transport includes buses, trams, metros and light rail, but excludes railways. London and Paris were excluded, as they both distort the national figures in the last column, as seems the case in Greece and Athens.)

Two points are concealed but underpin these statistics:

- 11 of the 19 large UK cities rely solely on buses. 7 had either trams or metros, and only London had 4 – bus, tube, light rail and a modest tram network. In mainland Europe, only 6 of the 57 large cities rely on buses, while 9 had three systems;
- all European cities retain some public control of their systems, although some outsource their services to private companies. In the UK, only 6 retain some control, though the picture is complex.

What the table shows is that the Netherlands and the UK make the fewest trips by urban transport. The Dutch make so many trips on foot and bike, while the British rely on cars. One has the most, the other the least, sustainable transport strategy in Europe.

Household emissions

As the IPCC states, no one can be left out, no household, no business, no government. Devolution should involve us all, however modest the difference. The average carbon footprint in the UK is about 7 tonnes per annum per person. In Germany, it is nearer 10 tonnes per annum, having retained most of its manufacturing sector. To anticipate the next chapter, so much British industry has either relocated to low-wage economies, or simply closed down.

To conclude this chapter on global warming, however, we turn to households, which account for about 18 per cent of UK emissions. These can be measured against the following eight consumer items.

1. electricity, 1 kWh = 1 kg CO_2,
2. gas, 1 m^3 = 2 kg CO_2,
3. petrol, oil and diesel, 1 litre = 2.5kg CO_2,
4. travel by bus, train, etc., 1 mile = 0.1 kg CO_2,
5. air travel, 1 hour = 150 kg CO_2,
6. food consumption, allow 900 kg CO_2 per person, and
7. for the public realm (industry, schools and hospitals, etc.), allow 900 kg per person, and

8. for consumables, allow 1,000 kg (1 tonne) CO_2 for every £15,000 of post-tax disposable income.

Concerning gas and electricity, better home insulation, draught exclusion and secondary glazing will reduce consumption. So would cooler indoor temperatures, as in previous decades, and wearing warmer clothes.

The average British driver averaged 1,230 trips and 10,300 miles each year from 1999–2001, while non-car owners survived on 750 trips and 2,750 miles a year (ONS; *Social Trends*, 2004). Assuming your car averages 10 miles/litre, your carbon emissions would reduce by at least 2.5 tonnes (or half that if you always have a passenger). Without a car, you might save £2,500 per annum in fuel, tax and insurance, recover some of those three wasted years of life in a non-productive haze, and rediscover more interesting or useful activities. In cities, excepting the disabled and specific trades, cars are an anti-social luxury.

You might not save money using public transport, but you would reduce emissions to 0.3 tonnes, and be able to work, read, meet strangers, relax or sleep.

With flying, don't! Unless it is essential. For those with private jets, like Philip Green who used to commute between London and Monaco most weekends, annual carbon emissions would be many thousands of tonnes.

You can reduce food emissions by eating what you buy, rather than letting a third of it go rotten or past its sell-by date, which is apparently the average household waste. You can grow much of your fruit and veg with a garden or allotment. Shopping in local shops and markets usually means less packaging, better value, and less food miles if you avoid non-seasonal imports like strawberries and... parsnips?

Despite arguing for increased spending on hospitals, industry and schools for example (see Chapters 1, 3 and 4), it is possible to make these investments while reducing carbon emissions. Thus, looking after your health would reduce hospital emissions, while local manufacturing reduces global transport and is usually more energy-efficient than in low-wage economies.

Finally, most consumables waste energy.

- A dishwasher uses 10–12 litres of very hot water per wash with very powerful detergents that dissolve glazes and bleach colours on most

china, while unable apparently to wash casserole dishes. It is possible to hand wash the same dishes with harmless detergents and 4–5 litres of hot water, plus rinsing water.
- Power and garden tools have replaced hand drills and push mowers, while clockwork seem to have disappeared. Perhaps wind-up clocks and watches require more metal and energy in manufacture, but battery clocks probably cost more in the long term.
- Even the humble tea bag wastes precious energy, grinding the tea leaves for the paper/plastic/glue bag, often in an envelope with a string, card and staple attached. It costs at least three times more per mug than a loose leaf brew, for an inferior drink.

The first five consumables above use energy directly, while all of them have varying degrees of 'embedded' energy in the production of machines, and in the infrastructure of roads, railways and national grids. Consumption can be moderated by pricing, as discussed for example with graduated gas and electricity prices (see Chapter 4).

Here, however, reducing personal emissions means altering our behaviour. In *Civilizing Cities*, I boast that my personal emissions are below three tonnes (and now nearer two with our Ukrainian 'squatter'). This is considerably lower than our friends in the comfortable classes. Of course I may be unusually tight-fisted, but our quality of life is little different to theirs in terms of comfort and convenience.

Yet however modest my carbon footprint, it is still considerably higher than perhaps 15 million UK citizens. 'Benefit scroungers' (as labelled by the Barclays, Murdoch and Rothermere) will have lower carbon footprints because they are often hungry or cold, only make essential trips and have no disposable income. It is the mindless wealthy (including those same media moguls) who are the scroungers: scrounging off the poor by paying minimum wages, scrounging off us all through tax evasion (ipE), scrounging bail-outs and tax allowances off the state, and scrounging off future generations by polluting the planet and wasting its resources.

In terms of strategy, to predict market demand for cars and then provide the necessary roads and car parks is unsustainable. To reduce transport energy consumption, we must reverse priorities in favour of bikes and pedestrians, emergency vehicles, public transport, local deliveries and last, non-essential car trips, with spending to match.

We must go further, however, and conserve all forms of energy (apart from muscle power), through tax and noise control, etc. We didn't hear one hand dryer in the Netherlands!

We used to regard water as inexhaustible. It isn't, and our attitude to energy is as foolhardy. Future generations will wonder how climate deniers, like Lee Raymond of ExxonMobil and the Koch Industry brothers, could be so powerful and prevent action to reduce carbon emissions. Yet the Exxon research team understood the risks its oil posed to global warming in the 1980s. According to Al Gore, such people are guilty of perhaps the greatest war crime since World War II. They are also hypocrites, arguing for small government while silent on their own malignant mega-corps – which undermine sustainable local economies, to which subject we now turn.

CHAPTER 3

Achieving a sustainable economy

A sustainable economy

The UK government has never defined what this means, relying instead on dogma and the GDP. The dogma is based on 'free-market' capitalism, in which the market is free of excessive 'red tape' and taxes, and business efficiency is measured by profit.

GDP (gross domestic product) measures the 'size' of an economy, simply by totalling all its financial transactions, not its efficiency or health. This is seriously misleading as it:

- excludes all voluntary and community activities, external costs like pollution, and fraudulent and corrupt transactions;
- ignores the inherent value of work, as 'quality' can't be measured, and unproductive 'dead' time, like commuting by car; and
- includes harmful and wasteful costs, like 'added value' (food adulteration and packaging), and the costs of tackling social problems. More crime requires more police, courts and prison wardens, thereby increasing GDP.

An extreme example comes from China. "When Chairman Mao once asked why farm crops had not met their five-year target, he was told that too many chaffinches were eating the corn. "Get rid of the chaffinches." Five years later, Mao asked the same question. With no chaffinches, plagues of insects were eating the crops. "Get rid of the insects." Five years later, crop targets were missed, this time because fruit crops failed. Bees are also insects. Today in parts of south China, small teams handpick pollen from the earlier flowering fruit trees and sell it to farmers back north to hand pollinate their trees. These new pollen gatherers and pollinators create either a positive increase in GDP... or an external cost of agrochemicals. Take your pick." (*Civilizing Cities*) Today's agrochemical mega-corps are little different.

Like traffic from the previous chapter, unregulated mega-corps disrupt our 'equilibrium with nature' with their excessive aviation, shipping and other 'external' costs. On the planet, nothing is external.

Our first true economist, Adam Smith (1723–1790), identified three sources of national wealth – Capital, Labour and Land – with Labour, and in particular its division into skills, creating most wealth. As argued in Chapters 4 and 5, that wealth is unfairly distributed and taxed to create and reinforce gross inequalities.

This chapter, however, must focus on the nature of business itself. Unfortunately, most governments understand business largely in terms of economics ('that dismal science') and its 'laws' of market forces, and supply and demand. But in every business and local economy, social interaction is as important as economic exchange. Even sole proprietors have to work with suppliers and customers.

Smith (who must be rescued from the neo-liberal grip of the Adam Smith Institute) understood this social nature of work. From his *Wealth of Nations*: "In civilized society, [man] stands at all times in need of the co-operation and assistance of great multitudes... [Like] no other living creature... man has almost constant occasion for the help of his brethren, and it is in vain for him to expect it from their benevolence only. [Every bargain] proposes to do this. Give me that which I want and you shall have this which you want... and it is in this manner that we obtain from one another the far greater part of those good offices which we stand in need of." Smith had stumbled on the biologists' evolutionary concept of 'reciprocal altruism' two centuries before R L Trivers in 1971.

Reciprocal altruism is the basis of our social nature – and healthy economies. Instead of getting the work/life balance 'right', work should be a central and rewarding part of our lives, alongside family, neighbourhood and political life. Today, however, with exported jobs, the gig economy, private equity, outsourced public services and boardroom greed, that fair bargain between Capital and Labour has broken down.

Before 1979, we enjoyed a mixed economy of private SMEs (small and medium-sized enterprises) and council public services, plus a few large companies and nationalized industries. Since then, our local economies have been monopolized by national and global mega-corps, local SMEs have been marginalized, and public services privatized by those solely in pursuit of profit. None of this is remotely sustainable – or healthy.

Covid and business

Before we turn to these three sectors – mega-corps, SMEs and the public sector – let Covid provide some European context and distinctly unflattering comparisons with the UK.

In the first six months of Covid, the UK GDP fell by 19.8 per cent compared with the European average of 11.4 per cent. (GDPs are useful for such comparisons.) Covid also introduced working from home (WFH). Mega-corps, with 'command management', could exploit this new concept, just as wealthy medieval wool merchants exploited families in this British 'cottage' industry. WFH denies the social nature of work, in which relaxed collaboration and humour usually underpin business innovation and efficiency, as well as personal health and social well-being. Together with the gig economy (with its minimum wages, zero hour contracts and no employment benefits), the UK job market is as challenging for young people as the housing market.

The UK also topped the emergency health spending. In that six months (March to September 2020), EU nations averaged €120 per capita. This ranged from €39 in the Netherlands and €50 in Denmark up to €274 in Ireland, €302 in Germany... and €446 in the UK (*Health at a Glance: Europe 2020*). And after two years, 2020/1 and 2021/2, estimates of UK emergency spending range from £311 billion or £4,631 per person (OBR), to £407 billion or £6,067 per person (IMF) (Brien and Keep: *Public spending during the Coronavirus-19 pandemic;* 2023. House of Commons Library).

Whatever the actual total, about a third of it was for business support. This included £45 billion available as small loans (up to £50,000) to nearly 2 million firms, of which at least £4.9 billion involved fraud due to 'schoolboy errors' and lack of 'due diligence' by the banks making the loans, which were guaranteed by the government. (*The Observer* 27/2/22).

Loans over €100 K, like our 'interruption loan schemes' for large firms, the EU insists should be made public. Post Brexit, our government has raised this bar to £500,000. Many think it should be £500. Secrecy makes an accurate assessment of value for money, including inefficiencies, profiteering and plain fraud, nigh impossible.

The furlough, or job retention, scheme, costing up to £14 billion a month, was also subject to fraud. Yet the police "will not routinely investigate or prioritise public sector fraud investigation at the expense of core business" (*Private Eye*, 1543). Either fraud is not serious, or the police, perhaps reasonably, thought that government contracts had safeguards against 'white-collar crime'.

Two other business problems – our reliance on global supply chains, and the poor value of privatized services – are discussed in the following relevant sections.

Mega-corps and the profit motive

Globalization emerged post-war with the World Bank and the IMF (International Monetary Fund), in which the US and other wealthy nations facilitated the interests of their own mega-corps through trade agreements, global finance and container transport. Unlike democracies, however, mega-corps are subject to minimal public scrutiny and regulatory control, thereby weakening all local and national economies. Instead of Adam Smith's market capitalism and free enterprise, where small firms operate in competitive local markets with modest profits, today's mega-corps have grown to dominate most business sectors. They share two basic features; profit focus and market share.

The right-wing economist and 'father of monetarism' Friedrich von Hayek (1899–1992), asserted that only the profit motive of the private sector can deliver efficiency. Public or government agencies are inherently socialist and inefficient. Despite strong evidence to the contrary (see later), the point here is that profit focus seriously distorts boardroom strategy. Maintaining high annual profits leads to short-term policies, reducing staff and production costs, and investing less in long-term R&D and risk management. Greater profits protect 'the financial interest of shareholders', which boardrooms see as their primary duty. Generous dividends are matched by the greed of directors and their accountants, bankers, consultants and lawyers. These rewards bear no relation to the wages of those who make the products or provide the services.

According to Smith, "the rate of profit does not, like rent and wages, rise with prosperity and fall with the declension of the society. On the contrary, it is naturally low in rich and high in poor countries, and it is always highest in the countries which are going fastest to ruin."

Yet mega-corps protect high profits through mergers and acquisitions of emerging competitors, creating oligopolies with over 15 per cent of market share. Tesco has over 30 per cent. With size, mega-corps become 'price makers' rather than small firm 'price takers'. (Perhaps 'price fixers' and 'price mixers' are more descriptive.) Mega-corp savings on labour and production costs usually inflate profits rather than reduce prices. Oligopolies may compete on price, usually to see how high they can be raised. During Covid, foodsheds, oil companies, energy suppliers and others increased prices when costs were largely static. This increased national inflation and created 'windfall' (unearned) profits.

The usual justification for size is that it brings 'economies of scale' and hence lower prices. But economies of scale peak among mid-sized companies, in accord with the Gaussian 'bell-shaped' curve of distribution. Beyond about 100 staff, higher transport costs, staff problems, bureaucracy and marketing create 'management drag'.

The economist Ronald Coase (1910–2013) had a different explanation. Large firms reduce 'transactional costs' by taking over their suppliers and buyers. But this denies the benefits of innovative and price-competitive SMEs, as discussed later.

Expanding market share (and profits) by acquiring emerging competitors is anti-competitive. In the UK, a handful of mega-corps (typically a 'big four') 'oligopolize' most employment sectors, from accountants and architects, banks and builders, chemicals and drugs, food manufacturers and foodsheds, buses and hauliers, energy suppliers, the media and oil companies, etc.

Consider the pharmaceutical mega-corp GSK (or to include all its major acquisitions from the Wikipedia profile, Glaxo-Affymax-Allen&Hanburys-Allergan-BeckmanInc-BeechamGroup-BlockDrug-BoroughsWellcome-CellZome-CNS-FrenchLaboratories-GlycoVaxyn-InternationalClinicalLaboratories-HumanGenomeSciences-JosephNathan-Kline&Co-LaboratoriosPhoenix-Maxinutrition-MeyerLaboratories-NordenLaboratories-PrestigeBrandsHoldings-RechercheetIndustrieTherapeutiques-Smith-StiefelLaboratories). Incorporating 24 independent 'pharmas' (some of them already mega-corps) reduces competition and diversity. It also reinforces skewed boardroom priorities. It seems that, as a company transforms from a product- or service-focussed SME to a profit-driven mega-corp, so corporate spending on marketing rises as investment in skills and R&D falls.

Pharmaceutical mega-corps invest less in research than in marketing. This often involves malpractice, like concealing research methodology and possible harmful side effects, and 'bribing' doctors and chemists to promote their drugs. Consider the potential of low-carb diets to reduce obesity and diabetes (from Chapter 1) and improve public health. Mega-corps, whether producing obesity drugs or junk foods (and 'ultra-processed foods') share the same profit focus. Increasing sales of junk food increases demand for obesity drugs. This presents the government with a conundrum. Fund the low-carb support groups through GPs, or continue buying the drugs. Over the next few years, the political lobbying and donations from the junk and drug peddlers must be monitored. With devolved primary healthcare, most councils would have no hesitation.

Coase also noted that mega-corps, by their very size, depend on 'command management'. The euphemism is 'incentivized' management, rewards going to those managers that exceed targets that are invariably profit-based. Improving products or staff conditions reduces short-term profits.

Mega-corps, like cattle that suffer 'hoove' from too much fodder, become bloated on excess profits extracted from local and national economies. Free of market regulation and engaging in price inflation, tax evasion in plain English (ipE), PR corruption and boardroom greed, mega-corps represent the survival of the fattest rather than the fittest. Corporate obesity is also unhealthy.

The Corporation documentary (2004) goes further. Mega-corps are psychopathic: they lie, show no concern for others, develop no long-term relationships, disregard safety, have no feelings of guilt and do not conform to social norms. Boardroom focus on profit and PR rather than product quality and staff motivation leads inevitably to lax risk control (with occasional catastrophic leaks and bangs like BP and Bhopal), market manipulation (such as price fixing and other illegal collusion), boardrooms divorced from shop floors (with high levels of sabotage concealed by high prices), anti-social behaviour toward customers and communities (ignoring the external costs of their operations), government influence (aka corruption) and evasion of justice (shareholders paying any fines while directors escape jail).

Mega-corps (with tourists) were also major Covid spreaders!

With profits and size come corporate power. 69 global mega-corps and 31 nations comprise the world's largest 100 economic entities. 'Globalization' is in fact today's neocolonialism. Snuffing out competition, reducing quality, exploiting staff and manipulating markets is ultimately only sustainable through force. Historic empires were built by the military and supported by transport infrastructure and finance. The Romans built roads for their legions, while Britain ruled the waves. Today's empire is based on unfair international trade agreements, free flow of capital and a global infrastructure that moves both capital and 40-tonne 'boxes' by sea, rail and road, with airfreight for lighter valuables and perishable goods.

The basic terms and conditions of these trade agreements enforce the mega-corps' 'right to trade' even over national environmental, employment or 'anti-competitive' laws. One exceptional case shed a singular ray of sunlight on this power. When the public water company of Cochabamba in Bolivia was sold to a private consortium led by Bechtel, it doubled the price of water and made the collecting of rainwater illegal. After three days of riots, the consortium pulled out. Later, it "filed suit against Bolivia for $25 million in losses. The claim was settled in 2006 for $0.30." (Wikipedia)

China is building its own empire.

Apparently, markets don't need a monopolies commission. Oligopolies are 'self-regulating'. Effectively, they are too big to fail. Rare failures, like Enron and Carillion, expose the collusion of their accountants, bankers and lawyers. What is clear from all textbooks is that excessive profits, size and secrecy undermine open, efficient and healthy markets – usually with government collusion.

If globalization emerged after 1945, **privatization** can be dated in the UK from 1979. Most of Europe was less committed, while most US public services were already privatized. First Thatcher sold most of the nationalized industries. Then Blair introduced private finance initiatives (PFIs) to build and manage public buildings and infrastructure, and since the Coalition, most public services have been outsourced. The profits of these private companies delivering public services demonstrate their greater 'efficiency' and allow gullible politicians to reduce public expenditure. But profits don't guarantee quality.

Consider the private water monopolies. Annual profits are substantial – and often illusory. For example, from 2007 to 2014, Thames Water (then owned by the Australian Macquarie Group) paid nearly £3 billion in dividends while increasing long-term debt from £1.6 billion to over £10 billion, and the pension deficit from £36 million to £249 million (*Private Eye* 1419). Not long after it took over, Macquarie advertised its major investment programme of over £1 billion per annum to upgrade the infrastructure. Insiders suggested that this was little more than its annual maintenance budget. Thames Water did gradually reduce leaking pipes, but continued to dump raw sewage in rivers during heavy rainfall due to grossly inadequate sewage treatment facilities.

Some of this sewage was noticed. From 2005 to 2013, Thames Water was fined £842,000 for 87 'events'. In 2016, there was a £1 million fine for one incident, and a year later, it was fined £20.3 million for dumping 1.5 billion litres of raw sewage in the Thames (Wikipedia). Yet these fines are derisory compared to annual dividends averaging £400 million. The fines being non-cumulative, it is cheaper to poison rivers and dump turds on beaches, and extract dividends rather than invest in proper treatment. The role of the regulator is marginal. But then, when the water boards were to be sold as private monopolies, a powerful regulator would have greatly reduced their sale price.

During Covid, the shortage of HGV drivers jeopardized the delivery of water treatment chemicals. So the private water monopolies sought permission to continue using rivers as sewers – without the fines. In 2021, the water companies admitted that they had dumped raw sewage into rivers and seas 372,544 times, for 2.6 million hours – though true figures may be higher. In the same year, the government kept no record of how many beaches had to be closed due to this sewage (*The Observer*, 6/11/22).

A proper regulator would have imposed on Thames Water a 3–5 year moratorium on dividends and bonuses, investing all profits in infrastructure improvements. Instead, Thames Water (through a 'separate company') was allowed to build a profitable multi-billion pounds 'super sewer' to cope with overflow during heavy rainfall. When it is complete, we will need a full income and expenditure statement by an independent auditor (excluding 'the big four' accountants) to assess value for money and integrity. As Thames Water users have to pay for it, we should know how our money was spent. A public water board would almost certainly have found, and indeed been expected to find, both cheaper and more sustainable solutions, like green roofs, porous surfaces in side streets and car parks, more domestic soakaways and upgraded sewage farms.

Few, if any, privatized public services can demonstrate improvements in the quality of service, user satisfaction, treatment of staff, environmental protection, value for money or public transparency. While the quality of public services delivered by local councils was variable, there was usually professional expertise and democratic control.

Private equity is the nadir of privatization. Private equity groups privatize public liability companies (PLC's) with huge loans, in effect converting corporate assets into debt, and taxable profits into loan repayments. The managers then reduce those loans, selling off capital assets, raising prices, reducing product or service quality and 'downsizing' staff and wages, except their own. Private equity enriches PLC shareholders, consultants, banks and the managers, at the expense of staff, customers, taxpayers and, eventually, the market when the company is refloated and collapses under its new debts. This is a negative-sum game.

Private equity has ravaged parts of the British economy. Consider the retail sector. Both Asda and Morrisons, two of the big four foodsheds, are now 'privatized'. When Morrisons was bought for £7 billion in 2021, within 18 months debt obligations of £3.2 billion rose to £7.5 billion when all debts were included. One common method of making private equity 'work' is to sell the valuable retail freeholds for substantial capital gains. Earlier, this had saddled the Debenhams chain with new expensive leasehold rents, forcing it to close about ten years later. Toys R Us, Maplin and HMV have suffered similar fates. Private equity involves buccaneering theft of capital assets and the closure of viable public businesses. All go back to the first private equity maverick, Hanson. Having bought the Allders department stores in 1983 and sold it ten years later, Allders went bust in 2005.

The government actually encourages this 'financial engineering'. Dividends (as 'unearned' income) are taxed at 8–39 per cent rather than 'earned' wage taxes rising from 20–45 per cent. And all corporate loan repayments are tax-exempt. The government makes no distinction between:

- loans that facilitate mega-corp mergers and acquisitions, thereby encouraging anti-competitive market manipulation with all the problems of size,
- debt repayments that private equity managers load onto companies like Thames Water and care homes, their anti-social profiteering at the expense of staff, suppliers, customers, taxpayers and the environment, and
- loans that facilitate internal expansion of existing firms which is healthy and should be tax deductible.

In summary, the libertarian ideology of unregulated capitalism has created anti-competitive global mega-corps. The wealth created is effectively privatized by the capitalists, largely at the expense of labour and quality. Mega-corps resemble monasteries from the Dark Ages. Secluded monks largely controlled religion with their monopoly of the Bible. Aloof boardroom executives largely control capitalism through their anti-social power over Capital, Labour – and governments. This contradicts the classical theory of economics. Big really is bad, as Adam Smith knew from the infamous East India Company. We now have a surfeit of East India Companies hoovering wealth out of all national economies, with the support of wealthy nations.

SMEs and the work ethic

SMEs, small and medium-sized enterprises, form the bedrock of every local economy. Every large town has, or had, thousands of them. All now are vulnerable as mega-corps expand.

The word 'ethic' may raise a few cynical eyebrows in this business context. "Ethic: 1 the principles of conduct governing an individual or a group: *professional ethics.* 2 a set of moral principles... " (*Penguin ED*). SMEs and mega-corps have very different work ethics.

- In SMEs, the principal focus is on product or service quality and staff motivation. Profits are essential for survival and success, but not the prime focus. Here the work ethic largely refers to group *principles* founded on professionalism.
- In mega-corps, the profit focus imposes boardroom decisions that too often flout moral principles of fair salaries, safe work conditions, risk safeguards and transparency, etc.

In general, SMEs are more efficient and democratic, with three specific advantages:

- their sheer number and diversity make local economies more resilient,
- they add substantially to social well-being, and
- they are more innovative.

When a large local firm or mega-corp plant goes bust, the local economy is seriously affected and recovery is slow. SME economies can survive the occasional failures, which are a symptom of a healthy economy. And local networking can often reduce such failures.

Social well-being is apparent with shops. In the UK, from 1971 to 2001, their number fell from 485,346 to 289,996 outlets (ONS), and is now likely to be well below 200,000. In 2002, the UK had 1.3 food shops per 1,000 people, the lowest in western Europe apart from Finland and Sweden. Germany had 2.1, France 2.2, Italy 3.9 and Spain the highest with 6.5 shops per 1,000. (Euromonitor: *European Marketing Data & Statistics, 2004*)

British foodsheds operate a *closed market*. They often pay small farmers less than the contract price, especially if the food is promoted in-store, design 'loss leaders' of staple foods like bread, beer and baked beans to close local shops rather than attract new shoppers, and frequently mislead customers with their promotions. Ethics?

Local shops operate in an *open market*, where wholesale markets ensure a fair price for the producers, the many shops giving a fair price to customers. Trust develops within this chain, in which shopkeepers and stallholders are the public face of the industry. After an hour spent shopping in a lively local centre, we return home enlivened by informal theatre, sharing information, personal anecdotes and jokes. In a foodshed, having filled the trolley, one swipes every barcode, then one's card before filling the boot, with no trace of human contact. I'm told it's worse than loading the dishwasher.

The 'discounters' showed just how expensive foodshed oligopolies were. Yet local shops and markets still sell fresh fruit and veg for less than half price, with friendly banter instead of foodshed packaging. In the best town centres, no foodshed can compete with independent bakers, butchers, cheese shops, fishmongers, health foods and fascinating delis (whether African, Chinese, Indian, Italian, Jewish, Polish and Turkish, etc.) that offer fascinating diversity with better price and quality on staples like cereals, olives and spices.

This compressed diversity of town centres is enriched with cafes, pubs and restaurants, cinemas and sports halls, offices and town halls – all threatened by out-of-town foodsheds, retail 'parks' and now e-commerce.

Innovative clusters are the third advantage of SMEs. Throughout Europe, many cities and regions developed manufacturing clusters. Britain could boast the Potteries (with 5,000 producers in its heyday, now reduced to about 2,000), Birmingham ('the engineering workshop of the world' but now much reduced) and Manchester the world's cotton capital, and now gone.

Jane Jacobs notes an MIT social scientist (Sabel) who, on the industrial clusters between Bologna and Venice in north Italy, "was amazed at the small size of these innovative and highly successful firms, most of which "employ from 5 to 50 workers, a few as many as 100, and a very few 250 or more... specializing in virtually every phase of the production of textiles, automatic machines, machine tools, automobiles, buses and agricultural equipment," and was impressed by the sophistication and quality of the work being done in production of ceramics, shoes, plastic furniture, motorcycles, woodcutting machinery, metal-cutting machinery, ceramics machinery. He reports the ease with which new enterprises have formed through break-away of workers from older enterprises, and the amazing economies of scale that are obtained not, as has been conventionally assumed, within the framework of huge organizations but rather through large symbiotic collections of little enterprises." (Jane Jacobs; *Cities and the Wealth of Nations*, 1984)

The UK created a new cluster in 1970, when Trinity college set up the Cambridge science park. By 1977, it had attracted 72 firms employing 3,500 people working in high-tech instruments, computer software, biotechnology and pharmaceuticals. In 2014, its website stated that it is the largest concentration of hi-tech enterprises in Europe, with over 100 firms employing "roughly 5,000 people in total". After nearly 40 years, the cluster confirms that SMEs, averaging about 50 staff per company, are key to successful innovation.

Clusters are not confined to industry. Many Italian Renaissance cities developed their own specialist clusters in art and architecture as well as manufacturing and banking. And while Haussmann was transforming Paris, Manet rescued French art from the dead hand of historical Classicism, leading to an explosion of 'art-isms' in the city's abundance of artists, studios, dealers and galleries.

SMEs, being owned, managed and staffed locally, are flexible and resilient. Their sheer numbers anchor, and specialist clusters strengthen local economies. They increase local skills and wages, develop local supply chains and specialist markets, circulate most turnover and profits locally, develop strategic links with universities and research institutes, and work as much by collaboration within their area as by competition with other clusters. This 'connectivity with the outside world' reinforces their social behaviour.

While profits remain essential for survival, the work ethic in clusters, as in social enterprises, is in product development and improvement, staff training and motivation, and creative collaboration within these 'symbiotic collections of little enterprises'. If personal reward were the prime motivator, then most of the Cambridge innovators would have quickly sold out to mega-corps, killing any cluster before it took root. By contrast, mega-corps destroy social interaction between shopfloor and boardroom through 'command management', and regard collaboration with suppliers and customers as 'transactional costs'.

To mega-corps, staff are their biggest cost; in clusters, staff are their biggest asset.

Among SMEs, there will be bad employers, but between the worst and the best, most will be decent, efficient and innovative, confirming yet again the bell-shaped curve of distribution. Working in SMEs can be an integral part of life with social value, personal motivation and economic rewards. And the impact of SMEs on the environment is modest, with no spectacular disasters.

During Covid, the purchase of PPE illustrates real European differences. Germany, Italy, Spain and Switzerland all centralized their purchasing of PPE. In the UK, having disrupted and downgraded the civil service since 2010, Hancock appointed Lord Deighton (a former Goldman Sachs banker) as PPE 'tsar'. He oversaw the award of multi-million pound Covid contracts to small private companies, many with minimal accounts, many just set up (like one of Hancock's local pub landlords) with no relevant expertise. Most had been recommended by 'friends' of MPs and their chums, political donors, accountants and government consultants. This whole farrago was dubbed a 'chumocracy' by our sniggering media, rather than plain corruption.

Expertise (and honesty) was rare. However speedy the delivery, more than 20 per cent of the PPE supplied did not actually meet the specifications. £2.9 billion of the stuff is unusable (*Private Eye* 1568). If expertise was rare, profiteering was rampant. From *Profits of Doom* (*Private Eye* 1560), just six individuals – Tim Horlick, Andrew Mills and Nathan Engelbrecht of Ayanda Capital, Banks Bourne of Tanner Pharma, David Meller of Meller Designs and Iain Liddell of the Uniserve group – apparently 'earned' commissions totalling £146 million. One modest public purchase might offer a fair comparison. The former MP for Wakefield, Imran Ahmad Khan (since imprisoned for serious sexual abuse) sourced 110,000 reusable face masks for the mid-Yorks hospital trust through an international charity and the Vietnam government.

Hancock assured us that most essential PPE would be sourced from British manufacturers. Local sourcing is vital, not only avoiding global supply chains and their excessive commissions and emissions, but also improving local resilience, with real social and economic benefits. Unfortunately, manufacturing has been marginalized since the 1980s when chancellor Lawson asked whether it was needed when our service sectors (including banks) were so strong.

One poignant example highlights this contrast between global and local. Rocialle Healthcare Ltd, with 75 staff in Girvan Ayrshire, was awarded £440 million to produce PPE. Jointly owned since 2019 by two (Australian and Chinese) medical product companies, it shared dividends of £50 million at the end of 2020. Then, in November 2021, the Girvan plant was shut and production moved to the Chinese parent company (*Private Eye* 1564). None of this is sustainable.

Of the 32 billion items of PPE bought by July 2020, only 8 per cent was manufactured in the UK, perhaps 8 per cent of PPE came direct from China, but most came via 'UK suppliers' above, themselves buying direct from China. To have excluded the public sector in the purchase of PPE was perverse.

Delivering public services

Most European nations retain a healthy public sector to manage schools and libraries, health and social services, energy and water supplies, public transport and law courts. Privatizers assert that, with market discipline, profit motivation and customer choice, private companies deliver those services more efficiently – and more cheaply. One can be rude about ideologues "... who have seized, or been seized by, an idea... but tended to lack an appreciation of the full script." (Joan Didion: *Miami*)

The T&T programme, the most ambitious public service contract during Covid, illuminated more of the script on privatization.

Briefly, by mid March 2021, PHE was overwhelmed trying to trace all contacts of those infected. So a new national programme was set up with a two-year budget of £37 billion. On 2nd April, Hancock promised that Covid tests would reach 100,000 a day by the end of April, with a new 'world-beating' T&T system under PHE, to be in place by 1st June. On 5th May, Baroness Dido Harding (another Tory peer, whose career was mostly in the boardrooms of Woolworths, Sainsbury's and TalkTalk) was appointed to lead PHE. She then appointed Mike Coupe, also from Sainsbury's, as her deputy to lead the Test element. Both elements were outsourced to private companies with little or no public health experience.

Deloitte (one of the 'big four' accountants and management consultants, but pretty poor at both) initially set up 42 drive-through testing sites. Most (subcontracted to Serco, Mitie, G4S, Sodexo and Boots) were in remote out-of-town car parks creating problems for all frontline staff in care homes and hospitals without a car. Central testing sites had to wait until August, but even in September, Harding had to apologize that many people's test appointments were still over a hundred miles (!) from where they lived.

The tests were then sent to one of three, later five, national laboratories. Allowing 24 hours for postal deliveries and 24 hours for lab analysis before sending the results to the national tracking system, local councils had to wait from three to seven days before they could contact those infected locally, some without postcodes, etc. The accuracy of the lab results also raised concerns. One large lab relied on low-paid lab assistants with tough 'efficiency' targets but lax protection against contaminated equipment falsifying results (BBC *Panorama*, 29/3/2021). Many local hospital and science labs could achieve reliable results within 24 hours of a test, but found it difficult to obtain equipment to increase their capacity. Effectively, they were ignored.

The national tracking programme was outsourced to Serco and the US call centre firm Sitel. Serco has dubious links to government, having been fined for fraudulently inflating fees on two previous public contracts – for which Deloitte, who happened to be their accountants, were also fined for not spotting the frauds. Both tracking firms lacked expertise and local presence. Predictably, tracking by low-paid staff from a few call centres with a national telephone line was inevitably poor. Many staff reported doing nothing for much of the time.

For the initial three month period, Serco and Sitel were paid £192 million. Yet during that same period, 76 per cent of the tracking (including all the 'complex' cases) was done by local public health teams who knew their areas, visited affected streets, advised residents and made crucial follow-up calls. They were given £300 million to cover this task. Even if that sum was only for the same three months (rather than the whole year), it indicates real value for money and quality of service from local councils that far outstrips the private companies.

Despite the large budget, T&T did not avert two further lockdowns, the third in January 2021. Setting up such a critical programme from scratch was bound to be challenging. But if the Covid inquiry is to compare the relative performance of the national private companies and local council teams, it needs full government disclosure on costs and KPIs (key performance indicators), PHE disclosing how the whole programme was managed and monitored, and the lead companies disclosing project management fees, use of subcontractors and profit levels, etc.

Without transparency, we can't compare corporate and council performance and value for money. But the official inquiry might assess actual performance against the following assertions:

- given the same resources, local councils would have delivered more test sites in convenient central locations, more quickly and cheaply than Deloitte;
- how the large test labs were selected needs to be reviewed, and their performance compared with that of small specialist research and hospital labs; and
- Serco and Sitel's tracking with a few national call centres were ineffective for many months, compared with the very efficient tracking

by local public health teams. Nor did they prevent two further lockdowns.

Outsourcing public services to the private sector is risky. Large private firms, led by strong-willed profit-driven amateurs, are not *de facto* more efficient delivering public contracts than experienced professionals in local councils, hospitals and research labs.

Whether T&T "was a good idea, or whether it worked, is above Serco's pay grade" as Rupert Soames of Serco modestly put it – on his pay in 2021 of £4.9 million. (*The Observer* 8/1/22) This suggests a disconnect between professional expertise and pay grade. If a corporate boss can't evaluate the value of T&T as delivered by his own firm, the Covid inquiry must do so.

The full script on privatization should include the lack of positive innovations and the many lamentable failures. Neo-conomists fail to see that competition and high salaries are not strong motivators in the public sector, except negatively when the dedication and expertise of frontline staff, whether nursing or teaching, etc., are valued at a small fraction of what aloof managers pay themselves for doing simple stress-free jobs. The 'public servant' is motivated by doing an important job well, and getting positive feedback from patients, pupils and parents, etc. In that, they are similar to shopkeepers and publicans. Even complaints can trigger innovation rather than dismissal, like the diabetic's complaint to her Southport GP (Chapter 1).

In effect, successful education facilities and primary healthcare services resemble SME clusters, co-ordinating and co-operating in their council area rather than competing to achieve what…?… cut costs, reduce expertise and, to maximize profits or reduce taxes, shut down 'failing' schools and care homes, and create local havoc? Councils are there to ensure that all facilities serve their purpose, with vital support services and funding for improvements.

Outsourcing public services raises another serious problem. Private firms only deliver what is specified in the contract. Any additional task leads to renegotiation of fees and significant cost creep. Yet all public services depend on flexibility managed by local experts. As its name suggests, privatization puts commercial confidentiality above contract transparency, personal greed above public need, and government control above local democracy. Yet privatization is now infecting education – see Chapter 4.

As local authority spending is regularly checked to ensure value for money, private firms should welcome the same discipline on all public contracts. As stated before, healthy markets require full disclosure for fair evaluation. Without it, we are denied the major benefit of hindsight. Secrecy covers up inefficiency, constricts choice, conceals excessive fees and corrodes public confidence.

Back in 1901, a comprehensive survey by Michigan University of all public services in the major cities of Europe and North America clearly revealed the whole script of private versus municipal (council) delivery of public services.

"The difficulties and limitations of comparison of private with municipal undertakings are numerous. In the first place, undertakings which are municipalized... have, in addition to the purely business side (profit and loss), an important social aspect; and municipal control means in almost every case a greater deal of attention paid to these social aspects, such as better facilities to the consuming public and better compensation to the employees. This amelioration of social conditions cannot be balanced in figures against diminished profits." (Fairlie, JA: *Municipal Administration*; Macmillan, 1901.)

Put bluntly, profit focus 'in almost every case' reduces staff salaries and service quality. Public agents deliver social value. History offers confirmation of Fairlie's conclusion. When Joseph Chamberlain municipalized Birmingham's three private gas companies in the 1870s, within five years, the gas works were improved, more homes were supplied, staff were paid more and gas prices were reduced – not once but twice (A Briggs, *Victorian Cities*). We might begin with our failing water companies, the railways, GP surgeries or...

Local mixed economies

"It's the creation of worth, not wealth, that's important." (J Garnett)

Sustainable economies maximize the local production of goods and delivery of services, with all local employers buying much more locally. The general strategy should be to replace 'imports' from mega-corps and encourage innovation (from Jacobs, *Cities and the Wealth of Nations*). Replacing global hoovers and private equity buccaneers with local SMEs and clusters would, as argued above, anchor local economies, reduce global emissions, increase local skills, and deliver public services under local democratic control.

This means reviving mixed economies in Britain, as in most of Europe. Whatever the government spends on business strategy, more should be spent on national regulators and business registers (see Chapter 5). Three former agencies, however, indicate the scope for devolving economic strategy:

- Business Links, from 1993 to 2011 as a national business counselling agency, was widely regarded as a waste of time, space and its annual budget of £105 million;
- also from the 1990s, the Manpower Services Commission was replaced by private Training and Enterprise Councils before morphing into Learning and Skills Councils in 2001 after concerns about TEC's financial probity (now being repeated with the Teesside freeport); and
- in 1998, the new Labour government set up regional development agencies (RDAs) to develop strategies and fund major projects in their areas. Councils had to compete for this public money. With an annual budget of c£2.25 billion, they were abolished in 2012.

Whatever a sustainable economy means, the best locus to develop and fund such strategies is in every council area, down among the business districts, industrial estates, workshops, farms, harbours, markets, high streets and colleges. Local chambers of trade and industry, in partnership with local councils and colleges, would be the best agents to produce

Achieving a sustainable economy

these strategies. They would reflect the diversity of each local economy and their different opportunities for growth and investment.

At present, British chambers are grossly underfunded. If membership was compulsory (as in France, with fees reflecting business size) and the government added a tenth of that RDA budget, the average chamber income would exceed £750,000 per annum, for small start-up grants, loans for SMEs and social enterprises, and training, etc. Chambers might even set up subregional investment banks jointly with neighbouring chambers. It's what local independent banks still do in Germany.

Consider how these local partnerships might support and develop farming. Although less than 1 per cent of GDP, it is a vital industry in many 'shire' economies, and part of our national heritage – or should be.

In 2020, the EU annual CAP budget (common agricultural policy) was about €55 billion, of which the UK received about £3.4 billion. If this level of subsidy is maintained, local sustainable strategies might include the following policies.

- Deliver all subsidies through local councils. MAFF or DEFRA (the government department responsible) was fined £647 million from 2005–2014, and another £230 million in 2015–2016 for failing to distribute EU subsidies to 80,000 English farmers on time (*Private Eye* 1452). Few councils would be so incompetent. The government only needs to set subsidy guidelines, whether as grants or loans. Each farming 'community' has very different needs for support, whether in livestock and dairy, cereals and cattle feed, horticulture and small-holdings, or mixed farming.
- Food security is essential. In 1981, we produced 405,000 tonnes of fruit (including soft fruit) from 60,000 hectares of orchards, while importing £1.72 billion of fruit and veg. In 2004, we only produced 283,000 tonnes of fruit from 33,000 hectares, while increasing imports to £4.92 billion (ONS). In 2002, France, Germany and Italy each produced roughly ten times as many apples (Euromonitor).
- UK milk production has spiralled into decline since the abolition of the Milk Marketing Board, producing about half of what is produced in France and Germany, with no protection against aggressive foodsheds.
- Farmers could protect local wildlife and the environment. Current government policy promoting environmental protection, however,

favours landowners over farmers – one of the main criticisms of CAP. Within a year of Brexit, the EU reformed CAP subsidies to focus on food production and smaller farms. (Before Brexit, apparently, it was the UK that resisted all attempts at such reform, happy to subsidize agro-businesses and wealthy landowners.)

- Food security need not contradict biodiversity. Organic farming protects the environment, but is less than 5 per cent of farmland, far lower than most nations in western Europe. 'Inorganic' farmers now spend over £3 billion per annum on fertilizers and pesticides that destroy natural habitats, kill wildlife, silence birdsong and poison rivers. Giving equivalent grants to double the saving on pesticides might encourage a much quicker conversion to organic farming. The lower yields/acre of organic crops emphasize the need to stop all greenfield development.
- Reducing the need for cattle feed would also release perhaps 40 per cent of arable farmland for more 'productive' crops. Returning cattle to natural pasture is also, apparently, as efficient as new woodland in storing carbon.
- We might also revive the recycling of waste food from restaurants to feed pigs and chickens, subject to the 'mad cow' disease or BSE (a sharp example of our disequilibrium with nature) that put a stop to the practice.
- Developing local food chains from farms and fishing ports to local markets, shops, schools and restaurants, would promote healthy fresh food and seasonal variety. This fair trade would release more farmers from unfair trade with the foodsheds and their unsustainable global food chains.
- Some might also reverse the dramatic loss of small abattoirs, caused by government veterinary charges that favour large abattoirs, and employ local vets rather than the current private monopoly sanctioned by the government.
- Some chambers might also, with grants or loans, support new food and drink manufacturers that 'add value' to local produce.

Any employment strategy must address two major challenges. Mega-corps must be reformed, perhaps on the model of the US *Sherman Antitrust Act* of 1890 to curb corporate power, by breaking them up into much smaller constituent firms, putting worker directors in the boardrooms (as in Germany and Japan), making directors personally responsible for their decisions, and prioritizing staff and product safety over the interests of shareholders. There is even a case for 'nationalizing' the drugs industry by funding all non-profit independent and university-based research institutes.

Second, we should focus on product and service quality, by putting the needs of SMEs above mega-corps, and reviving mixed economies. New chamber-council partnerships could develop the strengths of private enterprise and public expertise.

- The entrepreneurial skills of private sector SMEs provide goods and services under the discipline of 'market demand' rather than marketing. These skills are maximized in clusters of SMEs in town centres and science parks, etc., working as much in collaboration as in competition. Profit, essential for survival, is mostly re-invested locally in staff, property and research rather than extracted as dividends.
- The professional skills of the public sector deliver essential public goods and services under the discipline of 'cost control'. Here, delivering what we might call 'social demand' ensures that everyone enjoys basic human rights in a fair society. Thus, we might increase education services beyond school age, and increase public transport to reduce private traffic, but we should also try to *reduce* the social demand for hospital wards and prison wardens. The private sector is uncomfortable with this concept of 'reduced demand'.

Essentially, the private sector serves private needs for food and drink, clothes and shelter, plus desires for gadgets, fashion, toiletries and other fripperies. The public sector serves social needs for education, health and transport. The two sectors are complementary, and the innovative skills required, though different, are equally complex and compelling.

Problems emerge when 'market demand' creates social problems. Chapter 2 suggested that suburbs and cars, however popular, are unsustainable. Similarly, mega-corps, shamelessly exploiting junk foodies, gamblers and now vapers, resist the social need to control this 'market demand'.

This strategy of anti-trust regulation and reviving mixed economies contradicts the libertarian dogma of neo-conomists. Leaving us with powerful mega-corps that, in their 'bonding' with governments, may partly explain the rise of right-wing anti-social tyrannies throughout the globe – and neo-conomists.

Money is not neutral. Its value varies enormously. £10 spent in local shops and markets gives you far more fresh fruit and veg than in foodsheds, without the packaging and the cheating of farmers, but with some banter and a slightly stronger local economy. At the other extreme, £1 billion can buy you a few private jets and luxury yachts, or it can build several local libraries, primary schools and GP surgeries. Which of these strengthen local economies? And which, bringing us to the fourth principle for a sustainable future, improves social well-being and a just society?

CHAPTER 4

Ensuring a strong, healthy and just society

Social health

Health, in all its aspects, is the essence of life and the foundation for this whole recovery strategy. From previous chapters: personal health is at risk from underfunded health services; environmental health is polluted by policies that wilfully discriminate against energy-efficient modes of transport; and economic health is infected by mega-corps and privatization that impoverish local economies, putting private profits above social equity. Few of our European neighbours have sunk so low.

Thus, UK obesity affects 27 per cent of society, the highest in western Europe, where the average is 23 per cent (WHO *Regional Obesity Report* 2022). Similarly, our life expectancy is the lowest at 80.35 years, the highest being 83.21 in Norway (Wikipedia). This might simply reflect our lack of investment in public health and reliance on private cars, from chapters 1 and 2. However, there are alarming trends throughout the continent. While overweight people now average 59 per cent of European nations (and 64 per cent of the British), this has increased from 40 per cent in 1980. And for about ten years now, all Europeans' life expectancy has gone into decline. This probably reflects external factors (from Chapters 2 and 3), like anxiety over global warming and the powerful marketing of mega-corps.

Such measures of social health all demand a strong, healthy and just society, exposing a contradiction at the heart of British Conservative ideology. Macmillan's 'one nation Toryism' was swept aside in 1979 when Thatcher asserted that "There is no such thing as society; there are individual men and women, and there are families". Perhaps she thought that markets and neighbourhoods, work and pubs, sport and religion, protests and politics are just big families.

Her immature assertion founded a strident libertarianism, based on unregulated capitalism, low taxation and an indifference to human rights. Its lack of pragmatism, empathy and 'fair play' contradicts our national reputation and our nature as social animals. While poverty, apathy and anti-social behaviour create serious 'inefficiencies', so since 1979, successive Conservative governments have become increasingly intolerant, racist and inhumane. As Thomas Hobbes (1588–1679) wrote, without fair government, life for many becomes "solitary, poor, nasty, brutish, and short."

And society becomes weak, infirm and unjust.

During a national crisis, any government can expect general support from voters, even from opposition parties. "We're all in this together" is evidence of a strong society with mutual support and social solidarity. Covid exposed the contradiction between the mantra and reality. The British were not 'all in this together'.

- The wealthy were largely unaffected. Being unsocial, cocooned from street life by servants and chauffeurs in their excess of mansions and (untaxed) bedrooms, private yachts and jets, lockdowns were just another holiday.
- The comfortable classes, working from home (or a second home), were lonely or bored, and missed loved ones.
- The poor, key workers and ethnic minorities were 'all in this' and faced real stress. If infected, low-paid workers had to isolate for 14 days and go hungry. Home became a prison. If they continued working, just to survive, they were pilloried by the gutter press as 'plague carriers'. Lockdowns threatened their livelihoods.

Wealth and health are strongly correlated – excessive wealth inequality exacerbates health inequalities.

Let Laurence Sterne (1713–1768) provide our first positive definition of health. "O Blessed health! cried my father,... – thou art above all gold and treasure: 'tis thou who enlargest the soul, – and openist all its powers to receive instruction and to relish virtue. – He that has thee, has little more to wish for; – and he that is so wretched as to want thee, – wants every thing with thee." (*Tristram Shandy*, v. 5, ch. 33)

Few billionaires understand this. JM Keynes (writing in the 1930s) thought that millionaires needed psychiatrists rather than accountants to sort out their affairs. The wealthy are like 'junkies', airheads until their next deal. But while addicts largely damage only themselves, bling addicts inflict harm on society.

The New Zealand government understands this correlation between health and wealth, and the quality of lives and livelihoods. It focusses on general well-being and public health, rather than economic growth and GDP. It is difficult to be healthy when poor, unemployed, disabled, excluded or one of their children. With a fair balance between libertarian values and social fairness, social health emerges through fraternity, in clubs and neighbourhoods. Wealth is secondary.

The following text discusses first wealth inequality, as embedded by education, and health inequality with reference to housing. And as old people were the most vulnerable to Covid and ill health, it is the young who bear the brunt of inequality.

Wealth inequality

"Money works best when it's spread like manure." (Persian proverb)

The Spirit Level (Wilkinson and Pickett, 2010) is a fascinating study into income inequality among the wealthiest nations. In the most unequal societies (the UK, Portugal, the USA and Singapore) where the average household income of the top 20 per cent is at least seven times that of the bottom 20 per cent, social problems affect all levels of society. Even the wealthy suffer higher rates of infant mortality, teenage births, ill health, addiction, obesity, violent crime, prison sentences, stress and lack of trust, as well as fewer qualifications and a shorter lifespan than those in Japan and Scandinavia, the fairest societies with less than four times the income ratio. These nations are healthier with more social cohesion.

Before Covid, nearly six million British citizens received Universal Credit (UC). With Covid, Putin's invasion of Ukraine and inflation seriously increasing food and energy prices while reducing wages and benefits, poverty is now extreme and widespread. For 'the fifth largest economy in the world', unregulated capitalism is undermining society.

The poor do have banks, though food banks run by volunteers symbolize both social enterprise and innovation. The banks are now multi-banks, supplying basic essentials like kettles, clothes and bedding. Capitalism has also imposed time poverty on all those juggling two jobs to reduce the gap between minimum and living wages.

Fuel poverty affects all poor households. Following privatization, gas and electricity companies disconnected three times as many households as the former national boards. Unable to pay by direct debit, households then had to pay higher prices through pre-payment metres. No money meant no supply. British Gas even employed bailiffs to break into homes to install the metres. When does profit focus become psychopathic?

Smart companies could probably eliminate fuel poverty by graduating charges with their smart metres. A basic daily supply might be billed 'at cost' plus 10 per cent, with perhaps two higher bands doubling and trebling the cost per kWhr. This would also reduce excessive consumption, relieve pressure on power stations and might even increase profits.

Yet there is an ideological faith in ever-increasing consumption through 'market demand'. This highlights (from Chapter 3) the fault with GDP. Personal freedom is not an absolute. Energy, other than human muscle, is too precious to allow the wealthy to fritter it away on lawn mowers, leaf blowers, jets and yachts, when millions worry about boiling a kettle.

UK taxes too often discriminate in favour of wealth and power, notably on private transport and mega-corps, discussed further in Chapter 5. This discrimination also infected Chancellor Sunak's 'levelling up' funds to help councils recover from Covid.

Table 8. £220 million Community Renewal Fund in England, 2022

Local authorities	Councils	Projects	Total cost	Av/Project
Conservative councils:	30	134	£74,152,000	£553,373
Labour councils:	15	67	£38,434,000	£573,642
Other councils:	9	24	£12,725,000	£530,208

www.gov.uk

(The situation is more complicated in the other three nations, which account for the remaining £90 million of the programme.)

In England, figures for Conservative councils and projects exactly double the Labour figures. 20 of the Tory councils are shire counties, with 14 in the south of England.

The fund is part of the more ambitious £3.6 billion Towns Fund, to support local job creation in 101 'priority places'. Here 49 are Conservative-controlled, 42 Labour, 3 Lib-Dem, 4 Independent and 3 coalition. They include Richmond and Newark (Sunak's and Jenrick's constituencies) which are low on any index of multiple deprivation.

'Levelling up' is pure bluster. Government support continues to hit hardest those councils already the hardest hit. Yet sections of the press, particularly the Murdoch, Rothermere and Barclay 'comics', reported on the fear among 'blue wall' Tory councils that levelling up was at their expense. In contradicting the facts, they were patronizing voters in the new Tory 'red wall' constituencies, but meddling with the truth erodes democracy.

Government discrimination is at its most shameful when dealing with vulnerable minorities. The DWP outsourcing of disability benefits is inhumane. The Home Office 'hostile environment' to deport black British citizens is racist; its treatment of asylum seekers incomprehensible. Despite many serious labour shortages, exacerbated by Brexit, refugees are not allowed to work during their interminable and hostile review process. Stuck in mean hostels in remote areas, they can't even join local cricket teams. Ukrainian refugees were welcomed here, and hosts given £350 a month for 'rent'. Yet we couldn't host Syrians and Afghans, despite our obligations to the latter. Also, the government rent money was taken from the International Aid rather than Housing budget. Like transferring £5.5 billion from 'green' projects to building new roads (p. 37), this is indefensible.

This century, Europe has experienced extreme influxes of refugees from various conflicts in the middle east and north Africa. The Home Office ruthlessly targets hapless boat refugees from Calais that totalled about 43,000 in 2022, even as it gave visas to perhaps 550,000 immigrants in the same year. Since 2015, Germany has welcomed 1.7 million refugees from the Syrian crisis, 10,000 of whom have since gone to university there. "Wir schaffen das" ("We can do this") said Angela Merkel. We won't, even though our population growth during the 20th century was among the lowest in western Europe. Victorians would be ashamed by such hatred, but also bemused. They welcomed the poor and destitute, because they actually reinforced our prosperity. As a recent 50 pence coin put it, with sublime irony, "DIVERSITY BUILT BRITAIN". Racism as surely destroys it.

It is not too difficult to reduce wealth inequality through taxation, discussed in Chapter 5. Here, however, we need to understand the roots of unmerited wealth and poverty, which are embedded in our education system.

Education

"Education is correlated to most of the key life outcomes of an individual: employment, earnings, poverty levels, physical and mental health, well-being, social mobility, criminality and more." (OECD: *Equity and Quality in Education*; 2012)

As with health, however, UK state education is underfunded, over-controlled and now partly privatized. The following text briefly discusses the five stages of education; nursery (or early learning), primary and secondary schools, tertiary universities and colleges, and adult education.

If cars have denied children their first experience of social behaviour in streets, nursery schools were to socialize them in more formal settings. Yet with privatization and government cutbacks, increasingly nurseries are beyond the means of many families. One major initiative from Gordon Brown was the Sure Start family centres, set up in 1998 to offer all children 'the best possible start in life' through better childcare, early education, health and family support. By 2009, there were about 3,600 centres that in deprived areas, significantly improved children's health and 'cognitive development'. The centres had little impact in wealthy areas. Children nurtured in poverty suffer family stress, inactivity and lack of resources. Irrespective of their innate intelligence, poverty hinders their physical and mental development.

Government indifference to poverty contrasts with its control of primary and secondary schools. The national curriculum, SATs and Ofsted, PFI schools, academies and MATs have all reduced the concept of 'comprehensive education'.

Since 1991, primary schools have to follow a 'national curriculum', with two Key Stages for SATs (standard attainment tests). The narrow focus on English, maths and science, fatuously to better prepare children for work, creates real problems:

- the disproportionate emphasis on English and maths, marginalizes all other subjects or dispenses with them altogether;
- teachers are deluged every year with copious 'advisory notes' on how to teach these subjects. 'Teaching to the tests' ignores or over-rides many of their invaluable teaching skills; and
- the value of the core curriculum is dubious. One parent – a professional writer, helping her son during lockdown with his key stage 2 homework – found the English tasks incomprehensible and, in her words, 'joy squeezing'.

The national SATs target is to achieve an 80 per cent success rate in every school. Over-riding social variations between schools and regions is highly stressful. In many deprived areas, the target is an insult. In every school, teaching is seriously challenging, and compounded by gaps in learning, lack of resources and mental stress, exacerbated during Covid. Too many teachers leave within five years. Schools are like social enterprises; team effort, leadership, council resources and parental support ensure success, despite government interference. Having worked with a primary school that was almost bottom of the national 'league table', I would have happily sent our children there. Today, however, many parents move to the 'most successful' schools' catchment areas, based on those league tables, bringing class into every classroom and neighbourhood.

On top of SATs, the Blair government imposed Ofsted inspectors. While local councils still provide schools with relevant training, support and resources, none can prepare schools for a one-day inspection by an Ofsted inspector (sometimes without relevant experience) with a one or two word verdict; 'outstanding', 'good', 'inadequate' and 'special measures'.

This is plain abuse. Following the suicide of Ruth Perry, head of a school downgraded from outstanding to inadequate, the indefensible stress of these inspections demands proper scrutiny and reform. Recent ONS research suggests that nursery and primary teachers are 42 per cent more at risk of suicide than average. It is odd that the HSE (health and safety executive) doesn't automatically investigate all work-related suicides, as in France. But HSE funding has also been cut.

Before this mess of SATs, targets and Ofsted, most struggling schools received local council support services, advice and assistance, even sharing best practice with similar schools in a 'collegiate' manner based on mutual trust and empathy. The current system denies the importance of a comprehensive free-ranging education. Schools are not battery farms and children are not chickens. Nor indeed are teachers. Ofsted should not be disbanded, however, but re-directed to replace the incompetent Ofwat and Ofgen regulators and put the electricity, gas and water companies under 'special measures'.

After SATs came Blair's disastrous PFI (private finance initiative). This let private companies build new schools to be leased by local authorities as academies with exorbitant 'management fees'. Then, under the Coalition, education minister Gove and 'expert' Cummings put academies under direct government control, with more generous funding than schools remaining under council control. 'Freed from local council bureaucracy' (and expertise), academies were then 'herded' into MATs (multi academy trusts) with business leadership and management fees to match. Directors can earn over three times what council directors of education earn, while managing fewer schools. This inequality in MATs can lead to antagonism in staff rooms, less money for school resources and support services, and exacerbate demotivation.

Yet one of the largest MATs sheds light on the PFI. The boss of the United Learning Trust said that he would never take on another PFI school (*Private Eye* 1570).

The historic anomaly in education is private schools. In 2019/20, state schools spent just over £6,500/pupil, perhaps 10 per cent down in real terms from 2009/10, while facing inflation, rising costs and increasingly dilapidated buildings. Private schools have about £15,000 per annum for day pupils and £37,000 for each boarder. Unsurprisingly, with the best-paid teachers, smallest classes and best facilities, many private schools are among the top of the infamous school league tables, as measured by GCSE results. What is surprising is that many state schools are equally successful. It seems that the public sector *can* equal private schools, with less than 40 per cent of the funding.

Private schools enjoy a tax anomaly. Although profitable businesses, they have 'charitable status' and exemption from all corporate taxes. In effect, taxpayers subsidize the wealthy, whose children are not noticeably more intelligent than the mean. The schools then exploit this charitable status, offering 'scholarships' to those who can't afford the fees. In selecting the most intelligent pupils, at a stroke, they improve their exam results to the detriment of state schools.

About 7 per cent of pupils are privately educated. Yet they get well over 40 per cent of the top university places and a similar disproportion of top jobs among the 'ruling elite'; in legal chambers and the judiciary, in parliament and the civil service, in the media, the City and the banks. This sixfold advantage, based largely on privilege and self-confidence rather than merit, fitness and experience, reinforces wealth inequality. A self-perpetuating elite largely excluded from society in its formative years is hardly fit to govern that same society.

OECD comparative studies regularly confirm that a comprehensive system of education underpins a strong and fair society. "Stratification in school systems, which is the result of policies like grade repetition and selecting students at a young age for different 'tracks' or types of schools, is negatively related to equity; and students in highly stratified systems tend to be less motivated than those in less-stratified systems... Fairness in resource allocation is not only important for equity in education, but it is also related to the performance of the school system as a whole." (OECD: *PISA 2012 Results in Focus*; 2013)

All students need help to fulfil their potential, and also "to feel a sense of belonging both at school and in society" (OECD-Education International; *Principles for an Effective and Equitable Educational Recovery*; 2021).

During Covid, UK schools (like care homes) were left largely unprotected and closed during lockdowns, unlike Japan. The OECD report also noted that France had a 'well-developed digital learning infrastructure'. Many disadvantaged British students were without computers and thus excluded from remote learning.

The UK did introduce a 'catch-up tutoring' scheme to help those disadvantaged students, but the programme was flawed. Providing £300 million in its first year, with schools having to pay an extra 25 per cent fee for the tutors, one headteacher had "... one word for the tutoring plan: disastrous." (*The Observer*, 13/2/22) Apart from the 'byzantine complexity' of the government notes and website, few if any 'state' schools could afford the 25 per cent fees, so perhaps most tutors went to the more generously-funded MATs. (Did they actually pay the extra fees?)

Most of the funds, distributed through the Education Endowment Foundation (EEF), went to private firms. While EEF met its first year target, enrolling 250,000 pupils, the firms charged (up to) £90 per tutor hour, while paying tutors up to £40 an hour. As might be expected, many tutors were underqualified for their courses, were replaced during courses, or cancelled sessions at the last moment. (One firm reportedly 'employed' young online tutors from the far east at £1.50 an hour.) Tutors, like teachers, are undervalued and also scarce in many regions.

- If the tutoring scheme was indeed budgeted at £90 an hour, the whole £400 million fund should have provided nearly 4.5 million tutor hours.
- If local councils had managed the £400 million fund, paying tutors £35/hour plus £5 for management would have yielded 10 million tutor hours.

For the second year, against expectations, EEF was replaced by the Dutch mega-corp Randstad. From June to mid-December, 2021, it had enrolled pupils for 52,000 courses, against the target of 524,000 courses for the year. Such comparisons are essential to ensure value for money and accountability.

The risk now is that, during recovery, salaries will not return to pre-Bankers' Crash levels and more teachers will leave. And as the government ignored the risk of a pandemic, so it seems prepared to risk a serious school collapse or two, rather than restore capital spending to make all schools safe.

Outside school, too often we overlook 'children at risk' who are taken into care for their own protection. Removed to privatized care homes, these are often badly-managed, cold, even unsafe, and located where houses are cheapest rather than where the children live. "Some children were being moved to care homes more than 300 miles from their neighbourhoods.... A review by the Competition and Markets Authority last year found that the average operating profit per child in England was £45,000, with profit margins averaging 22.6%". (*The Observer*, 9/7/23)

The fourth largest provider, Outcomes First Group (owned by private equity firm Stirling Square), shut 28 of its homes early in 2023, of which at least seven were rated good or outstanding by Ofsted. What do "market challenges" mean when the group's profits rose from £3.5 million in 2020 to £5.5 million in 2021? (*The Observer*, 14/5/23) To repeat Adam Smith (from p. 32), "The rate of profit... is naturally low in rich and high in poor countries, and it is always highest in the countries which are going fastest to ruin." Are we rushing to ruin at the expense of our most vulnerable children?

Privatization is pervasive. Now universities are infected – sorry, 'incentivized'. According to Stiglitz, the best US universities are 'not-for-profit' enterprises. According to Malik, (*The Observer*, 18/3/2018) our universities lose intrinsic value "when managed as businesses, with students as customers and knowledge as a commodity." Instead of being centres of unfettered learning and research, universities are developing their own narrow version of the national curriculum, preparing students for work.

When students first had to pay their university fees in 2008, the annual government grant then was £3,000. When students were made responsible for all their university costs, in 2012, the Coalition also allowed universities to charge up to £9,000 annual fees – to create a market and introduce commercial discipline. Unsurprisingly, most charged the maximum, before embarking on expansion plans with top salaries to match. This created frequent discord between the new 'commercial' vice-chancellors and finance directors seeking to reduce costs, and lecturers and ancillary staff being 'casualized' and paid less. 'Market discipline' found that inferior impersonal online courses could replace lectures, reduce tuition costs and increase profits. When student numbers fell, 'underperforming' courses were cut, and lecturers 'downsized'.

For students, the situation is dire. Subsidized halls of residence became capital assets to be sold, the new owners charging students market rent. With an average student debt on graduation of over £45,000 and rising, each year about 300,000 graduates share a debt of £13.5 billion. These debts will affect them for 30–40 years, with the wealthier graduates repaying more quickly, and so less than lower-paid graduates like nurses and teachers. After ten years of managing the student loan 'business', total debt has reached £161 billion. This market isn't working.

The government is indifferent. For the Treasury, student loan repayments are a welcome 'cash cow'. If we treated education, like health, as a public service that is free from cradle to grave, how much would tertiary education cost if, as before, the government funded the universities and local councils paid student grants? With 1.87 million British students in 2019/20 (universitiesuk.ac.uk), allowing £10,000/student/annum (split perhaps equally between university fees and student grants) would cost taxpayers £19 billion per annum. Should taxpayers pay £190 billion over ten years to free young people of a substantial debt when they start their career, or is a cumulative debt of £161 billion over the same decade better? Economically, I don't know the full answer. I don't even understand the question. Socially, the first is fairer and more productive. The total cost to taxpayers could be reduced to perhaps £15 billion per annum if we means-tested the student grants. If we were mean, we might even insist that privately educated children should also pay their university costs!

A third group of vulnerable young people, after pre-school children living in poverty, and school children at risk of abuse, slip off the radar. 'NEETs' are those young people who have left school at 16, and 'disappear', some even denied the benefits to which they are entitled. The unfortunate moniker simply means 'not in education, employment or training'. Relevant social protection, health services, adequate housing and relevant training courses are seldom available to protect them from various social vices and the risks of 'grooming'. Herein lies a fruit of gross inequality. While the 'skills' of the privately educated elite, as stated earlier, are based on privilege and self-confidence, many teenagers facing privation have to develop basic survival skills and self-reliance in a hostile environment.

Health inequality and housing

Social injustice "is killing on a grand scale."

This was the general finding of the WHO Commission on Social Determinants of Health, 2007. The chair of that commission then produced the *Marmot Review on Health Equity* in England, when the government also enacted the *Child Poverty Act* 2010.

Ten years later, Marmot updated the *Review*. Under his five "social determinants of health", key findings over the last decade were as follows.

- "Give every child the best start in life." Poverty affects 30 per cent of children (or 4 million), putting us 29th of 37 OECD nations. We need to revive Sure Start and Children's Centres, improve maternity care and raise childcare pay.
- "Enable all children, young people and adults to maximise their capabilities and have control over their lives." Inequality remains in school results, and while pupil numbers and exclusions are both up, pupil funding is down 8 per cent, particularly in 6th forms and universities. Youth services are down 29 per cent, youth crime is up.
- "Create fair employment and good work for all." Zero hour contracts increased from 198,000 to 900,000, automation and work stress went up, while the quality of work and pay levels went down.
- "Ensure a healthy standard of living for all." While the wealth of the top decile was up 10 per cent, that of the bottom 30 per cent hardly changed. The UK is the most geographically unequal in Europe.
- "Create and develop healthy and sustainable places and communities." In the most deprived local authorities, net expenditure per resident was down 31 per cent. In the wealthiest councils, it was only down 16 per cent. So, following the Bankers' Crash and subsequent austerity, we were not all in this together.

If education embeds wealth inequality, housing reflects that inequality and seriously affects personal health and social justice. From billionaires' surplus mansions and yachts, comfortable class second homes, 'empty nesters' and the retired still in large family homes, Airbnb and holiday lets, we descend into landlords' extortionate market rents for flats, social housing denied adequate government funding, vulnerable groups in unfit houses, evicted families housed in 'temporary accommodation' and, off the 'housing ladder', the homeless.

Using the same five guiding principles, let us develop a green housing strategy.

Sound housing statistics. In a healthy housing market, supply meets demand. However, demand is complicated and divided between housing need and market demand.

- From ONS, the average annual population increase for England and Wales during the 1990s was about 140,000, 290,000 in the 2000s, and 400,000 in the last decade. With 2.3 persons in an average household, the annual demand rose from 65,000 to nearly 175,000 new homes.
- Without immigration, our population would be in steep decline due to emigration and falling birth rates. The British woman now bears an average 1.7 children against an average 2.1 children in developed nations, which is the level at which populations are stable.
- Demand from new households is probably in decline. While deaths of homeowners add to the supply, we now have the young leaving home much later, and often returning home after broken partnerships and/or lack of affordable homes.
- Against that decline, as households get smaller with more living alone or as childless couples, so demand rises for smaller homes.
- Market demand, as distinct for housing need, includes second homes, Airbnbs, holiday lets and empty 'investment vehicles'. (In areas with strong demand, these empty boxes, often 5 per cent of the total, benefit from annual price inflation of 8–10 per cent. Each new investment actually stokes price inflation and capital gains.)

The problems with supply are less confused. Today, the UK builds up to 200,000 new homes against a target of 300,000.

- We only built up to 300,000 in the 1960s, when councils were building nearly half of them. Since 1992, council housebuilding virtually ceased.
- Four large housebuilders dominate the supply. This is unhealthy. To maintain 25–30 per cent profit margins, they (and their banks) try to maintain high house prices – by restricting the supply?

- As between housing need and market demand, the government only requires the housebuilders to provide 'at least 10%' of their estates as affordable. This should be complemented by surtaxes on second homes and holiday lets, etc.
- The potential housing supply in long-vacant terraces, large under-occupied homes and vacant upper floors over shops is also ignored, see later.

At root, the national demand for homes is largely irrelevant. Many regions have a surplus. London and the southeast have too few. In 'tourism pressure areas' like Wales and the southwest, holiday homes displace many young people who can't afford to live where they were born and bred, only to find that almost everywhere, all young people have serious problems finding affordable homes.

Housing is first and foremost a local need, and, like public health and economic strategy, it needs to be managed locally.

Limiting environmental emissions. Housing accounts for nearly 20 per cent of UK carbon emissions (p. 30). This reflects housing density (see below) and building efficiency.

Assuming the same floorspace and external building materials, a suburban semi consumes about 50 per cent more energy than a terraced house, a bungalow twice as much. Terraces also have less 'embedded energy', conserving both land and building materials in their party walls.

Skyscrapers are also inefficient. While saving land, up to half of their bulk is underground, holding the building up. Above ground, the need for light material means glass walls, with excessive solar gain and winter heat loss. Reducing solar gain with tinted glass means office lights on all day, plus air conditioning as windows are impossible. And, unlike five- and six-storey buildings, lifts are in constant operation. All future skyscrapers should be turned on their side.

Disgracefully, unlike most of Europe, we have not improved the energy efficiency of new buildings. In 2006, the UK government determined that all new homes built from 2016 were to be energy neutral. In 2013, this deadline was deferred to 2025, see below.

Insulating existing homes would reduce carbon emissions much more quickly. Yet two government insulation schemes failed. The Green Deal programme from 2012, offering grants to home owners through a national agency and 20 national suppliers, was replaced in 2015 by the Home Insulation programme, through a handful of national builders. This was scrapped during Covid. Given those same funds, most local councils would have insulated more homes more quickly, more fairly by including social housing, and more cheaply by employing local builders and suppliers, thus strengthening local economies.

A sustainable construction industry must replace our centrifugal sprawl in search of an ersatz version of 'the American dream'. Compact towns and cities used to protect Britons from the extremes of climate. Today, suburban sprawl and exurban sheds have fuelled global warming and catastrophic weather events. Covering 14,000 sq. km of 'this green and pleasant land' is unsustainable, as discussed in Chapter 2, while suburbs may partly explain the 20th century rise in taking anti-depressants and sleeping pills, keeping pets and even talking to plants.

According to the *National Planning Policy Framework* (2012) "Sustainable development is about change for the better." This Panglossian view about 'progress' ignores a basic truth. Maintaining and adapting old buildings to suit current needs is inherently more sustainable than new green field development and brown field redevelopment. Slum clearance and now regeneration schemes destroy buildings often less than 50 years old. Yet all new construction is VAT-exempt while, inexplicably, all conservation work, repairing, insulating and extending existing buildings incurs 20 per cent VAT.

Most buildings should last centuries. The potential of vacant and underused buildings, plus small infill and backland developments, is enormous. In 2011, 750,000 homes (about 3.3 per cent of England's total stock) had been vacant for at least six months. It may be less now, but at least another 750,000 flats could be provided by converting large houses and vacant upper floors over shops.

Reusing old buildings conserves building materials, reduces global transport and releases all that construction energy and funding for more sustainable activities. Converted buildings also provide much cheaper premises for homes, business, leisure, social and civic uses. This benefits society by strengthening local economies and retaining local character and heritage.

Suburbs offer real potential to 'intensify' local areas. Consider a 1930s suburban centre with three-storey blocks of shops and cafes with flats above and rear service yards, plus a pub or two, served by a railway station and bus routes. Behind one block between two side streets, a dozen semis could be converted into 24 flats, or 36 with roof and rear extensions. More ambitiously, six pairs of adjacent semis could open up the generous back gardens with a lane between two small terraces, one of cottages, the other studio workshops with flats over. Such schemes for 12 semis could yield as many as 50 flats for young couples and social tenants, diversify the local area and strengthen local commerce and transport links.

A strong healthy society depends on maintaining neighbourhoods where social roots can develop in terraced streets with shops, pubs, schools and other social facilities fostering friendships sometimes over generations. Neighbourhoods take time to establish, but should last centuries.

In the last century, only the *Housing Act* 1969 supported stable neighbourhoods, replacing slum clearance with General Improvement Areas (GIAs) and home improvement grants as needed. Most GIA neighbourhoods remain to this day, but were scrapped after 1979. Perhaps they contradicted the interests of the powerful developers. Local builders were ignored.

The politics of continuity is cheaper, healthier, safer and more sustainable than 'the politics of change' that, since about 1900, has replaced social neighbourhoods with 'concrete jungles' and now urban renewal schemes. In these ghettoes, isolation and ennui are all-too-evident. They have also introduced such anti-social concepts as 'gated communities', 'poor doors' and even 'class cleansing', where developers ghettoize their schemes by paying for the affordable homes to be built elsewhere. Street life has largely disappeared, and inequality is built-in.

Covid reinforced that inequality. Stressed mortgage holders enjoyed a repayments holiday. Private renters, while protected against eviction, still had to pay their rents, even when furloughed on 80 per cent salaries. By November 2021, according to Citizens Advice, rent arrears had risen to £360 million. When evictions return, more people will become homeless or put in 'temporary accommodation' (*The Big Issue* 22/11/21).

The Chancellor did provide £750 million and £700 million to house the homeless – roughly double previous levels of support (*Private Eye* 1560).

Most was simply paid to empty hotel owners. For that same period, Sunak granted a Stamp duty 'holiday' on all house purchases up to £500,000 (over and above the £4 billion annual relief for first-time buyers). This indefensible subsidy of £7.6 billion gave comfortable homeowners up to £40,000 on each purchase, increasing house prices and second homes, and subsidizing the volume housebuilders, estate agents and private landlords (including, incidentally, many MPs). Had the Stamp duty been collected in both years, £7.6 billion would have allowed councils to house their homeless and, over time, reduce housing waiting lists.

Which leads us to **housing governance**. Three anecdotes illustrate government priorities. Having stopped council housebuilding, housing association subsidies are also reduced (see Table 9). They are encouraged to merge into ever-larger associations (like MATs, 'for efficiency'), and told to reduce rents – to reduce the cost of housing benefits. Inevitably, poor maintenance means families living in damp mouldy homes comparable to the worst private landlords.

Second, the deadline to make all new homes energy-neutral, mentioned earlier, was extended from 2016 to 2025 by Chancellor George Osborne, apparently after a lunch with Jeff Fairburn, then chief executive of housebuilder Persimmon. (I can't find the source for this anecdote, but include it because it is all too credible.) Resisting regulations that would reduce profit margins is common. But Persimmon also had more urgent priorities. After Fairburn was 'ousted' (with a 'severance' bonus of £108 million savagely reduced to £75 million), Persimmon had to focus on repairing serious faults that prevented many owners moving into their new jerry-built homes.

The other anecdote actually made the headlines. When Richard Desmond (former pornographer and newspaper owner turned property developer) dined with then minister Robert Jenrick, (at a 'fundraising' lunch that cost Desmond £12,000), he wanted speedy approval for a major housing development in Docklands to avoid the new 'community infrastructure levy' that would shortly affect all new development. This would have saved him about £40 million on a scheme costing well over £1 billion. The formal approval duly followed that lunch, until Jenricks' intervention was deemed illegal. The question here is not whether the Conservative party refunded Desmond's 'donation', but whether ministers should interfere with the local planning process that already has an independent appeal system in the Planning Inspectorate. All-too-often, ministers over-ride Inspectors' decisions.

Improving local schools and housing

Table 9 sets the financial context, and illustrates two points. While GDP is not a reliable guide to national prosperity (p. 55), it is invaluable to identify trends in spending on essential services as a percentage of GDP. And it confirms the absolute decline in public education and affordable housing post-1979, despite their revival under the Blair and Brown governments.

Table 9. Tax spending on education, health and housing 1982/3–2018/9 as percentage of GDP

Public service	1982/3	1988/9	1998/91	2008/9	2018/9
Education	5.39%	4.70%	4.51%	6.15%	4.31%
National health	5.16%	4.84%	5.49%	7.62%	7.49%
Housing	1.56%	0.81%	0.49%	1.22%	0.33%

ONS (www.statista.com for 2018/19)

However, the table conceals two serious trends. All tax spending on these vital services is increasingly spent by central government at the expense of local councils. This 'tax creep' has been ongoing for at least a century. In the 1930s, local councils spent 60–65 per cent of all tax revenue spending. This reduced to less than 50 per cent after the war due to nationalizing health, energy and water, about 30 per cent after outsourcing remaining public services, and is now about 20 per cent, after the Bankers' Crash and Osborne's austerity. This makes the UK the most centralized and perhaps the least democratic nation in western Europe.

And the outcome of these spending cuts since 2009 is largely ignored. Osborne's wilful austerity did not meet any financial objectives, national debt increasing from £1 tonne to £1.5 tonnes in 2016 and about £1.7 tonne now. It was also malicious in its social impact, particularly on children, the poor, social tenants and all public sector workers.

Consider the potential for devolution in education and housing, and how health and wealth inequalities should be reduced. Were education promoted, like health, as a free service available from cradle to grave, unlike the NHS, nursery, primary, secondary, college and adult education would be managed by LEAs (local education authorities), leaving universities with central government.

In 1990/1, central government funded nurseries, universities and vocational training, with 17 per cent of the total education budget. By 2007/8, it was 42 per cent, and continues to rise with the government's direct funding of the MATs, which now manage about 40 per cent of primary and 80 per cent of secondary schools. We need an independent inquiry to evaluate the performance of 'state' and 'free' schools, looking at value for money, financial probity and 'added value' as well as SATs.

Increasing funding significantly would enable LEAs to restore salaries of staff and those vital support services, and repair all school buildings to make them safe. (Shouldn't this essential remedial work on PFI schools be passed onto the owners of the buildings?)

More ambitious LEAs might emulate the success of ILEA (the inner London education authority), which enjoyed an international reputation for its educational achievements for such a mixed population from all backgrounds with so many languages. What teachers welcomed were the generous back-up services and facilities – language and diversity development, special needs and ed psychs, residential centres and trips, musical instruments and orchestras, sports facilities and digital infrastructure, etc. What the government didn't like was its high cost/pupil. ILEA was abolished in 1990.

Recovering from Covid also means addressing the following issues.

- The core curriculum needs to be much more flexible and appropriate. As an outsider, the English curriculum focusses primary schools on 'joy squeezing' grammar and syntax, when perhaps pupils should be

encouraged to 'express themselves' writing their own stories in their own way.
- Ofsted should be abolished. LEAs could carry out inspections on neighbouring LEAs to ensure some independence, while sharing examples of best practice.
- The benefits of digital learning are limited. The profit motive has no part to play in its use and it must not replace teachers and lecturers. Teaching, and group learning, is a social activity where, in effect, classes can resemble small social enterprises.
- Schools provide every child with their first formal introduction to social behaviour. They are also vital community hubs, and must be kept open in any future pandemic, with their playgrounds and sports fields protected against development.

For housing, local housing authorities are duty-bound to ensure that all residents are suitably housed. The clue is in their title. Most know better than central government just how serious and specific their local shortages are, yet lack the necessary powers and funding.

In 2007/8, councils spent £20.5 billion, mostly on housing benefits and 'temporary' (or emergency) accommodation in hostels and B&Bs that frequently last more than a year. The government spent £18.4 billion, partly on actually building houses in partnership with developers through unsustainable urban regeneration schemes. Seeing how it mismanages housing for the armed forces, outsourced to a private equity group based in the Channel Islands, it must leave housebuilding to local professionals under local democratic control, with their own mix of solutions.

Local builders, housing associations and co-ops might convert perhaps 25 per cent of the suburban semis occupied by retired couples, and vacant floors above shops into flats. Revived local rent tribunals would also protect tenants against excessive market rents. According to economist David Ricardo (1772–1823), "the interest of the landlord is always opposed to the interests of every other class in the community." And of course, we must tax mansions, second homes and empty 'investment boxes', as discussed in Chapter 5.

A strategy to reduce wealth inequality would focus on the relief of poverty, in part by corporate reform (Chapter 3) and by tax reform (Chapter 5).

Reducing health inequality was discussed in general terms in Chapter 1. Here, we might consider a specific strategy. To reduce obesity links all previous chapters: a serious health problem, exacerbated by motoring and marketing, that affects all wealthy nations. At root, the problem might resemble the Victorian problem with pubs, which attracted the poor, not only for the cheap gin and beer (safer than polluted water), but also for the light, warmth and social conviviality. Might our burger joints not serve a similar social function for the poor, as well as cheap junk food? Outlawing adverts to children, as well as promoting healthier diets and taxing harmful products, would perhaps reverse the continuing increase in obesity. A good government would at least attempt to reduce obesity.

Let me conclude with an alternative view of society to Thatcher's. In a science fiction classic, the hero asked the other four people ... " 'What's the answer?

"The robot bartender hurled its mixing glass across the room with a resounding crash. In the amazed silence that followed, Dagenham grunted: 'Damn! My radiation's disrupted your dolls again, Presteign.'

" 'The answer is yes,' the robot said, quite distinctly.

" 'What?' Foyle asked, taken aback.

" 'The answer to your question is yes.'

" 'Thank you,' Foyle said.

" 'My pleasure, sir,' the robot responded. 'A man is a member of society first, and an individual second. You must go along with society, whether it chooses destruction or not.' "

[Even if society is stupid?]... "Yes, sir, but you must teach society, not dictate.' "

Alfred Bester, even then (in *Tiger! Tiger!*, 1955), understood the difference between libertarian ideology and social democracy. The robot was wrong in one respect, however. We must now teach not society but our government about global destruction and social values, which brings us to the fifth and final guiding principle for *Securing our Future* – good governance.

CHAPTER 5

Promoting good governance

Politics is the basis of our social nature. A healthy democracy balances liberty and equality, letting us all lead our lives while ensuring that no one is without the basic essentials of life, from which emerges fraternity.

Today, Britain needs political leaders, at both the national and local levels, who combine intellectual rigour, social understanding and a felt need for fairness. Examples include Clement Attlee, Lloyd George and, in Birmingham, Joseph Chamberlain.

Since 1979, our governments have lacked these qualities, pursuing a 'right-wing' dogma of low taxes, corporate deregulation and privatization of public services, putting libertarian values above social equity. From previous chapters, governments have:

- invested less in our health services than all comparable nations, with negative impacts on staff, patients and general well-being;
- done little or nothing to prevent air and river pollution, protect natural habitats and reduce carbon emissions;
- actually encouraged anti-competitive mega-corps and anti-social private equity that reduce SMEs and weaken local economies; and
- endorsed shameful levels of wealth and health inequality.

To understand what 'a felt need for fairness' means, perhaps our most abstract science can help. Immanuel Kant (1724–1804) thought that we are all born with a sense of 'moral law'. *The Oxford Companion to Philosophy* (2001) clarifies his idea. "Moral judgements are expressions of practical as distinct from theoretical reason. Rather than taught/learnt from experience/by example, practical reason (including moral judgements) derives its principles from within its own rational nature." Perhaps, like Adam Smith, this is just another inkling of 'reciprocal altruism' (p. 56).

If moral judgement is innate (except in psychopaths who may lack this 'moral gene'), it can develop and mature to give us family life, social neighbourhoods, universal education, health care and welfare benefits. Unfortunately, nurture can also corrupt moral judgement. Imagine those brought up in dysfunctional families, then imprisoned in elite private schools before being pressed into vicious street gangs like the Bullingdonians. To these self-confident introverts, 'selfish by nurture', political integrity and social justice are meaningless, and power actively corrupts.

Having highlighted the imbalance between libertarian and social values in previous chapters, this may reflect successive governments' lack of moral judgement, but they were democratically elected. This final chapter discusses the failures not of policy but of 'governance' – 'the action or manner of governing or being governed' (*Penguin ED*).

Since 1979, successive UK governments have:

- centralized too much power and decision-making,
- neutered those 'checks and balances' that formerly curbed the worst excesses,
- ignored local expertise and eroded local democracy, relying instead on profit-driven amateurs to deliver public services,
- replaced public transparency with commercial confidentiality, frequent dishonesty and political corruption, and
- reduced taxes in favour of wealth, age and powerful elites, against poverty, the young, vulnerable minorities and public services.

These failures affect all areas of governance. All other Western European nations have retained stronger local government tiers, with more efficient public services, less privatization and significantly higher tax levels as a percentage of GDP (see below). This book can only offer an overview of our decline from a pragmatic 'fair-minded' democracy to an incompetent, corrupt and intolerant nation under dogmatic governments.

The following text divides the process of governing into five stages:

- understanding a problem,
- determining strategy,
- implementing policies,
- handling the finances, and
- reviewing outcomes.

All need fundamental reform.

Understanding a problem

Accurate, relevant and timely information is the basis for all strategy and policies. Three problems characterize this stage: the inadequacy of key national databases that protect privacy rather than transparency, the privatization of many government agencies that may corrupt independent research with commercial imperatives, and the failure to act on hard information.

This inertia was revealed by Covid. It was good governance for experts to test our state of readiness, following the Ebola and MERS outbreaks and WHO warnings about pandemics. The government understood the risks, and knew just how ill-prepared we were. Yet it ignored the strategic implications, concealed the findings of the Cygnus exercise, and then denied that even more relevant studies to Covid existed. Some policies, like outsourcing PPE and reducing hospital beds, actually magnified the risk. In effect, the government downgraded the risk, hoping that it wouldn't affect us, at least during this Parliament.

Mega-corps downgrade risk to increase profits, governments to reduce taxes. Both gamble with people's lives and livelihoods. Unfortunately, chickens come home to roost – occasionally with terrible consequences. Our government's cavalier approach caused well over 50,000 additional deaths. When Covid did arrive, if it had accurately recorded daily infections and deaths from the start, it would have grasped their gravity, imposed the first lockdown sooner and saved more thousands of lives.

Three national databases are crucial. The *Office for National Statistics* (ONS) provides an invaluable 'profile' every ten years on most aspects of life, with regular reports on key economic, social and environmental issues like inflation, pollution and crime, etc. It is not infallible. The 2011 national Census underestimated some local populations by more than 5 per cent. All censuses raise huge logistical difficulties, but this fault was entirely outside ONS control. 'Under-reporting' reflected fear among many British ethnic minorities, fuelled by the rise of UKIP, its anti-immigration policy following free movement within the EU after 2004, and the government's 'hostile environment' towards immigrants from 2010.

Local authorities found the discrepancies by comparing local ONS Census data with their school rolls, council taxpayers and electoral registers, etc. Statistics are most accurate at the local level.

Two other national databases lack the accuracy of the ONS. The *Land Registry* of property ownership covers less than 90 per cent of the land, and perhaps even less of all properties in England and Wales. Again, local authorities are more efficient at collecting council taxes based on properties than HMRC with personal and corporate taxes. In France, apparently, the true ownership of every field and building is not only recorded but is freely accessible to the public in every commune.

Similarly, *Companies House* records the business, financial accounts and directors of more than 4 million public and private enterprises (except building societies, charities and co-ops). At present, it is impossible to confirm the integrity and ownership of many companies. In fact, the government encourages secrecy.

- Limited liability partnerships (LLPs) were introduced to release partners, notably in the big four accountants, from personal liability for their often disastrous audits of large companies like Enron and Carillion. LLPs may largely account for the 34 per cent increase in Company House registrations from 2014 to 2020. From *Private Eye,* LLPs seem to be the vehicle of choice for money laundering, etc.
- Firms earning up to £10 million per annum are exempt from filing detailed annual accounts if they employ under 50 (?) staff. This threshold is far too high, and protects many dubious companies from public scrutiny, even on public contracts.
- Now, in tandem with the free flow of 'dirty money', Sunak is promoting free ports which will facilitate similar criminal activity in the import and export of goods – quite apart from the fraud endemic in the Teesside free port, according to *Private Eye* and now the *Financial Times.*

This lack of curiosity protects the UK as a tax haven, where dubious business activity is facilitated by accountants, bankers and lawyers. To be clear, government deregulation condones, and professional self-regulation conceals serious levels of national and global crime. Both Land Registry and Companies House must complete their databases with legal powers to enforce disclosure. The government even takes money from some of those criminals, laundered as political donations. This raises serious questions about the financial probity of the Conservative party and, in particular, some of its recent treasurers. All political parties must be rescued from the stink of corporate 'hospitality'.

Factual information and transparency are essential for democracy. Which brings us to **public messaging**. The two messengers are the government and the media.

The Statistics Act 2007 ensured that all scientific research and statistics were protected from persistent government meddling or 'spin'. Unfortunately, the Science Media Centre and other independent agencies that communicated on UK science were combined into UK Research and Innovation in 2018. "The move gave science a voice at No 10 and the Treasury but has also resulted in scientists losing independence and their own voice." (Fiona Fox, *The Observer*, 3/4/22) Truth and understanding are at risk when scientific news is refracted through government press teams.

Covid public messaging might have improved if SAGE had held separate press conferences, making it clear when the government followed the science, and when it deviated. Joint press briefings probably led both to shuffle towards a fudged compromise.

More seriously, the head of the UK Statistics Authority had to write to Hancock twice to correct his testing data in May/June 2020, and rebuke Johnson *several times* for claiming that more people were employed during Covid than before. Including the self employed, there were actually 600,000 fewer working. Too often, the government treated the crisis as an election campaign, boosting lies and half-truths. As with principles and partners, Johnson regards truth as a variable that depends on circumstance.

Most democracies treated their citizens as adults.

To be fair, government dishonesty is more widespread than we care to admit. In order to reduce unemployment figures, the relevant Thatcher department simply reclassified many of the unemployed as being 'disabled'. (Then, typically, many of those who had been reclassified were later exposed as 'benefit cheats' by the Rothermere, Barclay and Murdoch papers.) For Tony Blair, it was the Iraq dossier that 'justified' the illegal act of war and threatened the integrity of the BBC.

The media, for all their partisan faults, used to be an important check on government. Since Murdoch took over the *Sunday Times* in 1981, those faults have become systemic, as set out in Nick Davies' excellent, but depressing, *Flat Earth News*.

One of Murdoch's first acts was to disband the paper's Insight team, while retaining the brand. So instead of exposing the thalidomide tragedy and the Kim Philby scandal, we got the Hitler diaries, known to be a hoax before publication, Michael Foot exposed as a KGB spy before he successfully sued for libel, and its disgraceful coverage of the controversial *Death on the Rock* Thames TV documentary, the paper apparently rewriting copy from its own journalists in Gibraltar to bolster the government version of events.

When editor Andrew Neil retired in 1994, Murdoch congratulated him on "producing a paper that was three times bigger than under Harry Evans but with the same number of staff." Neil later wrote that: "On many of the biggest struggles of her decade in power, the *Sunday Times* stood shoulder to shoulder with her... Thatcher's battles were our battles." In this match of Thatcher's political convictions with Murdoch's financial ambition, the veto on cross-media ownership was quietly dropped. Murdoch's media empire now includes newspapers, TV, radio, books and films, where politics and profit corrupt journalistic integrity.

Maximizing profits means "not enough staff, not enough experience, not enough time" (Davies) to investigate stories properly and tell the truth to power. PR consultants outnumber journalists, major brands threaten to withdraw adverts in papers that have negative stories, and investigations now mean phone hacking and celebrity scoops, rather than the impact of privatizations. The Barclays have extracted so much profit from the *Telegraph* titles that they are no longer serious newspapers. Former porn baron Richard Desmond did the same to the *Express* papers, and Paul Dacre floods the *Mail* with his virulent suburban spleen.

British local newspapers (about 800) are not immune. Most are owned by 12 groups that close local offices and employ far fewer journalists in one or two remote 'hubs', who rely on the web for local news. Profits rely on adverts rather than scoops.

Public broadcasting is under threat. The Referendum damaged the BBC's reputation as it failed to 'balance' neo-political ignorance, dismissal of experts and loud jingoistic soundbites (aka Nigel Farage) with facts and rational analysis. By appointing Richard Sharp as BBC chairman (a Tory party donor, ex Goldman Sachs banker, former boss of Rishi Sunak, member of the right-wing think tank Centre for Policy Research and facilitator of an £800,000 loan for then prime minister Johnson), alongside (former Tory council candidate) Tim Davie as director general, the government was only repeating Blair's imposition of two Labour sympathisers, Gavyn Davies and Greg Dyke, as BBC chair and director general. Then, however, the BBC broadcast its scoop on the Iraq dossier that led to the illegal war. (The unsatisfactory Hutton Inquiry into the affair exonerated the government, but then judicial inquiries have a marked tendency to exonerate any government involved. The current Covid inquiry may well be exceptional in this regard.)

The BBC's latest problem was exposed by another footballer, this time ex-player Gary Lineker. Having compared the racist language of Suella Braverman's policies about refugees in small boats to 1930s Nazi Germany, Sharp and Davie sought to remove him from *Match of the Day*. Instead of broadcasters holding governments to account, governments threaten their independence. However, Sharp and Davie then discovered that most BBC staff had the same sense of 'moral law'.

BBC and Channel Four's attempts to remain impartial, protect truth and challenge power, however naïve, contrast with the 'social platforms' that protect 'freedom of speech' for all users. The consequent lies and hate, inciting violence, homophobia, misogyny, racism and religious intolerance with occasional mass killings and war crimes, surely *demand* regulation. Platform owners must edit content to protect basic truths, and employ US workers to do this hugely stressful work, rather than outsource it to low-paid workers in poor nations. Then, gradually by 'word of mouth', fellow citizens might appreciate the personal traumas, social damage and the necessity for regulation. While China controls social platforms to indoctrinate citizens and enforce conformity, US owners of Facebook and Twitter, etc. 'mine' their platforms solely to maximize profits. Both rely on cant rather than Kant's moral judgement. These anti-social platforms are dragging us all into a new Dark Age where tyranny and genocide thrive.

Determining strategy

Since 1979, governments have pursued few long-term strategies. Thatcher (or Tina – 'There is no alternative') curbed the unions ('the enemy within'), unleashed market forces on planning, and reduced taxes. Blair emphasized education with increased funding (Table 9) but undermined it by increasing government control, imposing PFI schools, SATs and Ofsted. Since Cameron, we have ideologues without relevant expertise devising strategy: education (Gove's special advisor Dominic Cummings), public health (led by retail director Dido Harding), the T&T programme (managed by accountants and call centres), and 'Brexit – led by donkeys', confirmed by Gove's contempt for experts during the referendum.

Consider four strategies: regulation, Brexit, the economy and a sustainable future. Regulation is a basic function of governance. Since 1979, regulations covering most business activity have been relaxed or withdrawn, with little assessment of possible impacts. Three examples, while rewarding the few, led to huge social costs.

The Big Bang of 1983 deregulated the Stock Exchange, allowing large banks, British and foreign, to expand into all financial sectors. As with all mega-corps, scrutiny and curbs on anti-competitive behaviour is difficult, and impossible when governments support those businesses. Many now admit what some foresaw: the Big Bang eventually boomeranged, with banking excesses landing us all with the Bankers' Crash. Belatedly, the *Financial Conduct Authority* (FCA) was founded in 2013, but it is too weak to moderate let alone reform the banking system.

As with banks, so with privatized industries. The private water monopolies have been illegally dumping raw sewage into our rivers and on our beaches with impunity (see Chapter 3). In May 2023, they finally apologized and promised to address this major catastrophe – by raising prices! Imagine what public water companies would have done with £72 billion that the water companies have extracted as dividends since 1990, plus the bonuses paid to board directors. Before nationalization and then privatization, most of our water was under municipal control, as it remains in Germany. As suggested above, private water companies should be placed under 'special measures', with a moratorium on dividends and bonuses for several years so that all profits are invested in essential infrastructure and reducing debt burdens.

Major developers and housebuilders also resisted regulations to improve building energy efficiency (from Chapter 4). Ironically, improving tower block insulation led to the Grenfell disaster because the cladding material was highly flammable. The relevant government department and ministers, the (privatized) Building Research Establishment, the materials manufacturer, building contractors, and the Kensington and Chelsea borough and TMO (tenant management organization) were all criminally negligent in ignoring previous fires in buildings clad with similar materials. Ignorance is no excuse.

Saving a few hundred million pounds in the many buildings so clad killed 72 Grenfell residents, and traumatized hundreds of their relatives and neighbours. Cynics might argue, again misusing the concept of 'common sense', that at least the building industry and GDP will benefit from the several billion pounds needed to remedy what was clearly a tragedy foretold. This GDP boost is doubly negative, however, as it imprisons many thousands of residents living in all blocks of flats with similar cladding, fearful yet unable to sell their property, and possibly having to pay some of the costs of insurance, fire protection and remedial works.

Perhaps MPs who publicly promote further deregulation should have 'Grenfell' or 'Sewage' tattooed on their foreheads.

Which brings us to Brexit and 'taking back control'. We don't know precisely which EU regulations, affecting employment rights, environmental safeguards, water standards, financial services and building regulations, etc., the former Brexit minister Jacob Rees-Mogg wanted to cancel.

Brexit illustrates the huge damage that results from major decisions made without a strategy. It is the worst decision made since the war, combining the arrogance of Cameron and Osborne with the ignorance of Johnson and Farage, whose lies and deceits were cruelly exposed by Covid.

That £350 million a week promised to the NHS (roughly £17.5 billion per annum) was never going to happen. Much of it was actually lost to fraud in the various business support programmes.

Taking back control so far has meant exports to Europe down 14 per cent in the last quarter of 2021 compared with two years previously, and all investment down. The small trade deals with Australia and New Zealand actually cede control of UK (and EU) farming standards that will put many British farms at risk or out of business.

This act of incalculable self-harm denies the UK access to a civilized union with so many joint initiatives, scientific projects, social benefits, personal freedoms, cultural exchanges, environmental standards, legal safeguards and a large open market with so many opportunities for young people. Like the impact of long Covid on people, the economic and social consequences of Brexit will be far-reaching and long-lasting.

Widely unremarked is that, since Brexit, the Northern Ireland economy has actually performed better than the rest of the UK. After the initial shock of staff shortages and disrupted food chains, Northern Ireland fairly quickly replaced most internal UK trade with £1 billion of extra unhampered trade with the rest of Ireland, plus increased trade with the wider EU. Manufacturing jobs also grew faster than in the rest of the UK (*The Observer*, 15/5/22). Ferry traffic from Northern Ireland to Great Britain declined by 50 per cent, traffic direct to Europe increased 400 per cent.

Unfortunately, access to real statistics, accurate media reporting and common sense are in short supply. There was one beam of light. After Johnson's 'oven-ready' EU treaty threatened the Northern Ireland Protocol and the very future of the UK, Sunak negotiated an honest and impressive deal with the EU. Promoting the deal to the DUP in Northern Ireland, he actually said this. "If we get the executive [in Stormont] up and running, Northern Ireland is in the unbelievably special position... in having privileged access not just to the UK home market (which is the 5th biggest in the world), but also the European Union single market. Nobody else has that. No one." Great Britain should follow suit. However, with duplicity and fear infecting both main parties, political sanity will be delayed.

Outside Europe, Johnson posed two strategies. 'Levelling up' was ignored (p. 82/3), and replaced with 'a high skills, high wage and low tax economy'. Like most political soundbites, this offered a superficial gloss. High skills in specialist clusters are increasingly vulnerable in Britain, to both mega-corps and now Brexit. Instead of open access to the large and progressive European free trade market (which Thatcher was instrumental in introducing), exporters suddenly exposed to border chaos must find new global markets, open EU subsidiaries, relocate there or go bust.

High wages depend on these specialist clusters. In a few low-paid jobs, like HGV drivers, wages are now more commensurate with the skills and dedication involved. But the loss of seasonal workers and skilled Europeans post-Brexit leaves us with serious labour shortages in many sectors (and crops left to rot in fields) not experienced elsewhere in Europe. Here, high wages are concentrated in boardrooms, at the expense of 'shopfloor' staff in care homes and hospitals, schools and universities, shops, pubs and hotels, in private equity firms, outsourced public services, the gig economy and even, regrettably, in local councils. Almost all sectors suffer job losses or depressed wages. Wealth creation has become a 'zero sum game'. Europe offers the best potential for high skills and high wages, particularly for young people.

Yet when a genuine demand for 'high' wages emerges, the government resists. Following ten years of austerity and then Brexit, the UK has seen an unprecedented wave of strikes by highly skilled workers in the public sector. After the trauma of Covid, teachers and lecturers, bus drivers, post and railway workers, ambulance drivers and paramedics, nurses and doctors have all held strikes, for better pay, working conditions and essential resources. This far exceeded the 'winter of discontent' of 1978/9, for which Callaghan was held directly responsible ("Crisis? What crisis?"). Today it's the workers rather than Sunak. Both governments sought to impose wage restraint to reduce inflation. This blunt tool ignores more significant factors, notably unjustified price hikes by profiteering firms (shown by their subsequent inflated profits) and serious inflation of earnings above £150,000.

Union leaders generally face negative media. Thus, ambulance drivers and nurses were always asked about 'the likely increased deaths' caused by their strikes. Rarely came the clear response "We've been killing patients for years because we have insufficient staff, beds and resources – but you've not noticed." Almost every pre-Covid BBC *Hospital* programme included at least one cancellation of a vital long-overdue operation. No one exposed the government's cavalier attitude to patient safety and staff exhaustion.

Also overlooked, the strikes were rigorously managed, as required by various post-1979 reforms to 'regulate' union activities. The official ballots of members, often achieving over 80 per cent voting in favour of strikes in essential services, demonstrated democracy in action. Public servants and society deserve better.

Finally, the government declines to define sustainability in its own 'strategy for a sustainable future', relying on the Brundtland definition: "development that meets the needs of the present without compromising the ability of future generations to meet their now needs." This is unsatisfactory.

Philosophers are more helpful. Edmund Burke (1729–1797) thought that society is a contract or "... partnership not only between those who are living, but between those who are living, those who are dead, and those who are to be born." John Stuart Mill (1806–1873) emphasized this continuity with the past. "The best government [is that which gives people] that for want of which they cannot advance, or advance only in a lame and lopsided manner. We must not, however, forget the reservation necessary in all things which have for their object improvement, or Progress; namely, that in seeking the good which is needed, no damage, or as little as possible, be done to that already possessed." Summarizing Mill a century later, Karl Popper(1902–1994) would restrict all political and social progress to "small-scale incrementalism".

A sustainable strategy rooted in the past, and seeking physical, economic and social improvements, requires the following:

- maximize the conservation of existing buildings and infrastructure, and retain the local diversity of neighbourhoods, institutions and businesses;
- meet the needs of all citizens through small-scale urban intensification, provide affordable housing, primary healthcare, expansive education and training, and invest in the local production of goods and services; and
- protect future generations from the known hazards of pollution, depletion of finite resources, and destruction of natural habitats and biodiversity.

This replaces 'the [fatuous] politics of change' with continuity, committing us to progressive incremental changes towards social justice, environmental protection and economic equity. The risk is that, the longer we delay essential policies to mitigate the crisis, the more desperate the remedies required.

One shining example was Major's introduction of the 'fuel escalator'. In the face of a few motorists' protests, the Brown government dropped the escalator. Then Cameron reintroduced it – but on train fares rather than petrol. Sunak retained the fares escalator, but actually reduced fuel duties. Which brings us to implementation.

Implementing policies

Privatization comes into its own when implementing policies. First, the government sold its own agencies. Within the justice department, for example, the Courts Translation Service, National Forensic Laboratories and Probation Service were privatized. With translators and forensics, concerns are that, in maximizing profits, less well-paid translators may be insufficiently qualified, or lab technicians may have less time for complex cases, leading occasionally to unsafe verdicts. Probation has recently been 're-nationalized'.

Other national laboratories, like the Building Research Establishment, the Food and Environment Research Agency, Qineteq (formerly Defence Evaluation and Research Agency) and the Transport Research Laboratory have also been sold. Most public research agencies are more 'open-minded' in their work, and worrying that ownership of private laboratories is not always clear.

Government confidence in private companies is the inverse of its contempt for public expertise. This may derive from the unmerited self-confidence that is the defining hallmark of private school inmates (or out-patients?). Contempt also characterized the governments of Hitler and Stalin, one arrogantly replacing his generals, the other insanely suspicious of them.

Policy implementation has two basic stages: ministers first assess policy alternatives with civil servants, and then select the best agencies to implement them. Government policy was a compromise between ministers' manifesto promises, and civil service expertise in 'governance', with non-political judgement that ensures vital continuity and checks against extreme or unworkable policies.

Government contempt may have originated in a historical civil service fault of patronizing aloofness, but post-1979, it was their lack of 'commercial nous' in managing privatizations. Three policies weakened the service:

- under Thatcher, it was 'strengthened' with an influx of business managers to provide that commercial perspective,
- following spending reviews in 2010 and 2015, 470,000 civil servants were reduced by 20 per cent. Although numbers are now back to 2010 levels following Brexit and Covid, disgracefully HMRC is still 10 per cent under-strength, and
- ministers now often bypass their servants and go to commercial 'experts'.

Instead of civil servants bullying their hapless ministers with 'passive aggression' (according to Dominic Raab's experience), ministers employ pliable management consultants. These are not cheap. Deloitte, EY, KPMG, McKinsey and PwC charge from £1,000 to £6,000 a day, about ten times what junior and senior civil servants are paid. The spectacular Carillion and Enron bankruptcies suggest that these experts either don't understand such large businesses or, for such large fees, they collude with management. Either way, they confirm a serious habit with all consultants, simply confirming what clients want to hear. Thus they colluded in the ruinous school and hospital PFI (private finance initiative) contracts, providing figures based on assumptions that even GCSE economic students would have seen through. Occasionally the penny drops, as when one MAT refuses to 'rescue' any PFI school (p. 86).

A major weakness of the civil service (identified by Lord Crowther-Hunt in the mid 1970s) is that professional experts in each civil service department are subservient to generalist administrators. Now the service has become increasingly 'politicized' with little appreciation of the dangers involved.

The US manages this core aspect of governance far better. From Michael Lewis' *The Fifth Risk,* all government departments give their political administrators and 'entrepreneurs' equal status rather than hierarchy. The latter innovate in areas of public interest, like public safety or sustainability, that have no commercial potential to exploit, or where commercial exploitation needs to be improved or regulated.

Historically, implementing policies was usually left to local councils, where most public services originated. The only public services that require central management are foreign policy and national defence. All other public services require local (and/or regional) management and delivery. Or used to. Central control of these local services is inefficient and undemocratic: inefficient because imposing an ideological "one size fits all" policy may be irrelevant or counter-productive in very different localities; undemocratic because it forbids different approaches by local councils and experts. One size never fits all.

This erosion of local government has a long history. *Civilizing Cities* identifies three key dates.

"In 1871, with local council powers at their height, the Local Government Board was set up. According to Sir Robert Ensor (*OEH* 1988), "it is difficult to over-estimate what the country lost through having its local authorities down to 1914 placed under a central department constantly on the alert to hinder them and rarely, if ever, to help. The much greater progress made by Prussia between 1870 and 1914 on many sides of local government administration was associated with an almost opposite relation between centre and circumference"...

"Following 1945, many municipal services were nationalized... Here, the fault lay not in the *principle* of public services, but in their management by unelected regional authorities, national boards and government departments. This disenfranchised local councils and local democratic control ceased.

"Finally, from 1979, most remaining council services were privatized along with the nationalized industries: [including refuse collection under 'compulsory competitive tender', internal council services outsourced, municipal bus companies sold off, independent MAT schools imposed, and council houses sold to private landlords].

"Councils are no longer 'supreme in their own sphere of jurisdiction'. When Margaret Thatcher called for the return of Victorian values, she over-shot her target, reviving a neo-Georgian era of private privilege, naked profiteering and political indifference to poverty and public squalor. We have replaced public services with commercial contracts, quality control with performance targets, value for money with private profits and democratic control with commercial confidentiality."

There is also a legal impediment. Local councils are only allowed (and obliged) to do what Parliament decrees. All other action is *ultra vires*, outside their powers and illegal.

Covid demonstrated this contempt. The government defined our understanding of the problem, our strategic response, policy implementation and funding. Local authorities were largely bypassed except as lockdown agents. A 'local authority' has become an oxymoron – without power. The government decides all public strategy, before telling local councils how to implement those services or ordering them to be outsourced.

The ambitious £37 billion T&T (test and track) programme was delivered by remote profit-driven strong-willed amateurs, rather than by councils with their public health expertise, collective experience and local infrastructure. Corporate managers had to grasp the complexities and outcomes of the public contract, determine the best approach and required staff numbers, qualifications and resources and then, the tricky bit, employ those teams while ensuring handsome profits – their prime duty apparently being to maximize the interest of shareholders. This breezy replacement of local experts by remote amateurs negates the principles of 'using sound science responsibly' and of 'good governance'.

Most public services have been removed from meaningful local democratic control – even in planning. We need to revive the Victorians' 'municipal gospel' and restore local government spending to the levels of the 1930s so that they can deliver fully those services that the law requires of them – and more.

Such drastic reduction of local government is unknown in most of Europe, and even the US. Privatization is now ingrained in most public services. Cynics suggest a barely-concealed strategy – to so reduce funding, service quality and staff morale in hospitals, schools and local councils that the public will accept further privatization.

The underlying danger is that, instead of government controlling mega-corps, they have infiltrated government and largely control strategy and policy in their own interests. All government/private partnerships tend to corrupt. Now governments – Tory and Labour – begin to behave like mega-corps. Both increasingly control public services, at the expense of public service staff and users.

If Jesus expelled moneylenders from temples, so we must expel mega-corps, lobby groups and PR from the corridors of power. The stink of corruption is pervasive.

Raising taxes

All nations tax wealth to pay for universal public services like education, health and transport, and provide basic welfare for all. Perhaps wealth inequality and the difference between libertarian values and social equity is best illustrated in national tax revenues.

In 2020, the UK tax burden, at 33.3 per cent of GDP, was *almost* the lowest in western Europe:

- all 26 nations above the UK were in Europe (apart from Cuba 40.6 per cent), including Spain, Germany, Italy and Scandinavia, rising to France at 46.2 per cent of GDP;
- from 30–33 per cent were Brazil, Canada, New Zealand and Japan;
- below 30 per cent were the US 27.1 per cent, Russia 24.2 per cent, Ireland 22.8 per cent, India 18.1 per cent and China 17.5 per cent;
- at the bottom were the Middle East oil tyrannies with taxes less than 5 per cent of GDP (Wikipedia).

Table 10. UK government tax income £m, 2007/8

Income tax	144,443 (27.7% of total)
National insurance (NI)	95,437 (18.3%)
• employers' contr'n	54,030
• employees' contr'n	39,250
• self employed	3,032
VAT	92,433 (17.8%)
Duties, etc.	64,434 (12.4%)
• Fuel duty	24,905
• Stamp duty	14,123
Corporation tax	46,383 (8.9%)
Council tax	23,637 (4.5%)
Non domestic rates	19,584 (3.8%)
All other income	34,263 (6.6%)
Total	520,614 (100%)

Source: ONS

Table 10 identifies the main tax revenues. With austerity since 2008, excess spending on Covid and inflation, these figures have changed. In 2019, total tax was £620 billion, but the proportions broadly persist. Thus, NI (national insurance) fell from 18.3 per cent of the total to 17.5 per cent in 2019, but may well rise again.

The following is an idiot's guide to taxation (possibly written by one) in part to counter the needless complexity of the system. In fact, this very complexity may be designed to confuse and deter public scrutiny. So, accepting that tax can only be raised on wealth, it is possible to apportion these taxes, however approximately, against Adam Smith's three sources of wealth; namely Labour (income), Capital (investment) and Land (and property), as follows:

- Labour pays perhaps £372.8 billion, or 72 per cent of the total, through income tax and NI, 90 per cent of the VAT and all duties except the Stamp duty. £372.8 billion is roughly 43% of total earnings in 2007/8 of £870 billion;

- Capital, through Corporation tax and 10 per cent of VAT, paid £55.6 billion or nearly 11 per cent;
- Land, through Stamp duty, Council tax and Business rates, paid £57.3 billion or 11 per cent of total tax revenue.

Smith thought that Labour, and in particular the division of labour, created most wealth. Today, mechanization, property speculation and e-technology may have reduced labour's contribution. The proposed tax reforms below are based on three broad assumptions.

First, to reduce wealth inequality, Labour's share of the tax burden could be reduced to 60 per cent or less, with Capital and Land sharing the rest. The government partly agrees. To strengthen public finances after Covid; "The fairest way to continue to fund excellent public services is with the highest-earning households contributing more, and companies contributing in recognition of the support they have received from the government." (HM Treasury, *Budget 2021*) Land and property were ignored.

Second, we must increase total tax revenues over time by perhaps 20 per cent if we are to meet the ever-increasing demand for those 'excellent [?] public services' since at least 1900, and to make good the progressive underfunding since 1979.

Third, we must collect the taxes. According to HMRC, 'lost tax revenues' in 2011/2 totalled £40 billion, which could rise to £47 billion in 2014/5. This may well result from the needless complexity. Yet HMRC is still 10 per cent smaller than under previous governments.

All figures below are from ONS, and refer to 2007/8 unless otherwise stated.

a) Labour

Income tax was 16.6 per cent of total earnings of £870 billion. Increasing it to 20 per cent of earnings would have raised an extra £30 billion. This is not difficult, but first we must reduce income tax on the lower paid.

Eleven million workers earning less than £14,000 paid £6.9 billion in tax. This was 6.3 per cent of their total earnings of £108.8 billion, or perhaps 10 per cent after excluding those earning less than the tax threshold. We could raise the tax threshold to the 'living wage' level, or re-introduce the

10 per cent tax rate on earnings above the minimum wage to say £20,000 pa. These would reduce total tax revenue by perhaps £10 billion.

To increase income tax revenue, we must first increase the tax on high earners. The 192,000 workers earning over £200,000 paid 34.5 per cent (£32.4 billion) of their £93.9 billion total earnings. Increasing this to 50 per cent would raise at least £15 billion extra revenue, with possible tax bands as follows:

- on income above 10x the minimum wage (roughly the prime minister's wage of £125,000), it should be 50 per cent,
- on income 80x the minimum wage (about £1 million per annum) it should be 80 per cent, with intermediate rises.

Second, income from Capital and Land, as dividends and rents, is taxed as 'unearned' rather than earned income. This tax distinction, one of the few honest descriptions to emerge from the Treasury, doesn't explain why dividends are taxed from 8.75–39.35 per cent over £150,000. It penalizes the hard sweat of Labour over the restful sleep of Capital and Land. Taxing all income equally would increase revenue by perhaps £10 billion. Philip Green (?) once tried to justify this indulgence because the wealthy put their own money at risk. Comparing financial and physical risk, like working on fishing boats and building sites, or in chemical plants, hospitals and prisons, is absurd.

Third, most personal tax allowances simply protect unearned wealth. It would be fairer and more efficient to treat all welfare benefits as basic rights, available on receipt of a doctor's or job centre's note. And remove every other tax allowance apart from the universal personal, family and age allowances. The formerly 'non-domicile' residents of 11 and now 10 Downing Street avoided tax bills of as much as £20 million – perfectly legally. Some wealthy people apparently claim their offshore bank withdrawals as non-taxable loans rather than income. And that tax relief on chauffeurs (can it still be true?) mocks all disabled people who've had their mobility allowances reduced or withdrawn by underqualified staff underpaid by profiteering employers.

b) Capital

First corporation tax must be collected. Corporate 'tax efficiency' or courtroom 'tax avoidance' is actually tax evasion in plain English, or fraud. Simplest would be to tax all companies, large and small, on their UK revenues, as before 1965. Even accountants would have difficulty fiddling turnover figures. A revenue tax graduated like income tax would curb the anti-competitive growth of mega-corps and oligopolies more effectively than any monopolies commission. It would also share in the 'windfall' profits of the oil companies, energy suppliers and foodsheds when prices surged following the invasion of Ukraine.

Bill Gates suggested a tax on technology, noting that workers are taxed on their income, but machines doing the same job are not. This subsidizes Capital at the expense of Labour. Perhaps employers should pay all NI, on the workers who have been taught and trained at public expense, and on machines to reflect their external costs of energy consumption, noise and unemployment.

Finally, we need a bonfire not of corporate red tape, but of their tax allowances. This includes tax relief on loans that subsidize mega-corps' monopolistic growth and private equity financial engineers (Chapter 3).

c) Land

Land and property, the third source of personal wealth, are subject to Stamp duty when bought, capital gains when sold and inheritance tax when the owner dies. All need to be collected.

- When the 6th Duke of Westminster died in 2016, his eldest son inherited the whole estate, valued at some £9 billion, tax-free via an offshore family trust. Tax should be levied on every property and landholding, irrespective of where the deeds are kept.
- Also in 2016, research showed that landowners received £13 billion tax-free when they sold their land for exurban development (*The Planner*, September 2018). In Germany, local councils first identify *and buy* the land needed for urban growth, and then invite tenders from developers. This retains most of the enhanced land value for the public good rather than the landowners.

- Farms (of which the largest farm owner is James Dyson) are apparently exempt from inheritance tax, despite benefiting from the various farm and environmental subsidies.

Stamp duty on property is difficult to evade. Currently, it rises to 12 per cent on English properties over £1.5 million. Were 12 per cent the average, revenue would double. In 2008, this would have raised £15 billion (when the top rate was only 8 per cent). Buyers of multi-million pound properties might bleat at 25 per cent, but most would be paid by the owner/developers due to lower prices. As house prices principally reflect 'public demand', it is only fair that some of that value returns to the public.

Both the council tax and business 'rates' must be reformed. The former, based on 1991 (!) house prices, is absurd. A £50 million central London mansion pays less tax than a £320,000 home in any other city because, both being in the top price band H and all houses in central London in band H, those boroughs can set the lowest council tax rates. They prefer to lower the tax rather than provide and maintain social housing in their areas – witness Grenfell tower.

If the average home is valued at £300,000, the aggregate value of 27 million homes is about £8 trillion. Replacing the council tax with an annual graduated home tax of 1 per cent (as in Denmark) would raise £80 billion. If commercial property were included, this new property tax could well exceed £120 billion per annum, at least doubling the existing council tax and business rates.

This property tax might 'level up' George Osborne's innovative (or vindictive) bedroom tax on social tenants. A modest tax on second bedrooms would ensure that most pay this replacement for the council tax, with additional bedrooms taxed progressively. Alternatively, basing the tax on floor area would penalize basement cinemas and swimming pools more fairly. Either way, second homes should be included.

The only caveat to any property or wealth tax is that it should be collected centrally, to benefit from the gross wealth of central London boroughs and the corrupt anomaly that is the City of London, before distributing it fairly to all local authorities.

Value Added Tax

VAT is imposed on most of our purchases, but also on all stages of production, from raw materials to components, product assembly, packaging and sale. It has at least three flaws:

- it seems to be a second tax on Labour that has already paid income tax and NI when supplying those same goods and services;
- the wealthy evade it, buying their jets and yachts in tax havens. Perhaps we should just surtax them whenever they berth or land in British ports; and
- VAT makes no distinction between new and recycled goods. So repairing domestic appliances and commercial goods is often more expensive than replacing with new. 'Built-in obsolescence' is unsustainable technology. Perversely, as discussed in Chapter 3, new buildings are VAT-exempt while building maintenance and extensions pay 20 per cent. Urban intensification and local builders are penalized to protect excessive profits of the national housebuilders and developers.

Replacing VAT with a luxury or value reduced tax (VRT) would curb pollution, waste and consumerism, conserve materials and energy, and possibly redirect GDP to more positive activities.

The fuel duty is such a VRT. Had the escalator continued from 2008, revenues would have doubled by now. With tax relief on all low incomes, making the fuel duty 'tax neutral', this would have benefited the poor and other non-car owners. A parking tax might also raise perhaps £5 billion for its wasteful use of land.

VRT should also apply to oil companies. "The left-of-centre think tank Common Wealth found that Shell and BP have channelled £147bn to shareholders via dividends and share buybacks over the past decade, with rival North Sea producers and the big six energy suppliers contributing another £47bn." (*The Observer*, 31/10/21 and 6/2/22) Instead, BP and Shell enjoy tax rebates on North Sea oil and gas production.

Finally, advertising should incur VRT, as it reduces social value, increases prices, violates the young and encourages excessive consumption. Its underbelly, public relations or PR, is anything but public, corrupting the media, politics and honest public discourse. Taxing adverts would also put a brake on the obscene profits of the anti-social platforms.

Some hoped that during Covid, the government might address some of the worst tax anomalies that favour bankers, hedge funds, private equity, landlords and billionaires at the expense of honest workers, the low paid, young people, the disabled, refugees and all who depend on welfare benefits. However, given ministers' own personal wealth, backgrounds and political donors (aka friends), honest reform was unlikely. Some tax changes actually reinforced these disparities.

There is another serious problem, namely in managing tax spending. Largely due to privatization, all government spending on infrastructure projects, defence contracts and outsourced services suffers from chronic cost creep, as discussed in Chapter 2 on highway costs and HS2. In European business circles we are known as 'Treasure Island'. This is embarrassing. To the cynic, it is probably as well that our government spending is only 33 per cent of GDP. Consider how it would mislay, misspend and misappropriate 46 per cent as in France.

Major crises create extreme challenges that usually require economic 'solutions'. During the Bankers' Crash, the Bank of England printed about £500 billion of new money. This 'quantitative easing' (QE) was 'injected' into the economy by buying government bonds to shore up confidence in the stock market, and encourage banks to start lending again. Protecting those who own such assets meant that much or most of the QE simply enriched wealthy investors 'riding' the market. Bailing out the banks without imposing reforms left our high street banks (and us) tied to the casino banks and their gambling.

During Covid, the total emergency QE was between £310 billion and £410 billion, (p. 57). Perhaps half of this went into business support schemes and through outsourced public service contracts like T&T and PPE purchase.

Future injections of QE must include local councils, either directly from the government or from the Bank via the Public Works Loan Board. With Covid, most councils would have focussed on public health rather than profit, and delivered PPE, T&T and support for local firms more efficiently with a better grip on finance. During the Bankers' Crash, councils might have invested that QE in vital public service improvements, long-delayed infrastructure projects and local charities, reviving local economies and relieving those most in need.

Delivering most public services through local councils is more democratic. With their local expertise, infrastructure and transparent audits, most offer real value for money. It is better to have a few rogue councils that can be dealt with, rather than one centralized government that displays serious levels of incompetence and corruption. Effective devolution would revive some sense of local authority, upon which local democracy depends.

We need to think local. And act local.

Reviewing outcomes

Government reform presents a conundrum. Good governance avoids the need for reform, bad governance denies that need. To rescue us from this slough of despond, we need local and national politicians gifted with social awareness, intellectual rigour and a felt need for fairness. History offers Joseph Chamberlain for his municipal transformation of Birmingham in the 1870s, Lloyd George with national insurance and state pensions, Clement Attlee for the NHS, British Rail and legal aid, etc., and Harold Wilson for various social reforms, the Open University and refusing to join the US in Vietnam. These reforms improved social life for all, while curbing the excessive power and profits of the few. In short, balancing Liberty and Equality more fairly encouraged Fraternity.

Since 1979, the whole landscape of UK governance changed. Democracy has become a two-tier process between government and citizens – those who govern and those who are governed. In elections of the 1960s, Quentin Hogg (later Lord Hailsham) frequently warned us that "a vote for Labour is a vote for elective dictatorship". Few of us then understood what he meant. Now we know. Our decline since 1979 displays clear symptoms of 'elective dictatorship'.

- All democracies have three tiers, national, local (or regional) and citizens. Our local councils are largely bypassed, essential public services now outsourced to profit-driven amateurs. This dogmatic aversion affects all public sector experts, so civil servants are bullied or replaced by pliable consultants.
- Privatization has created unhealthy partnerships between government and mega-corps, with their consultants, trade lobbies, PR and secondments infecting government strategy. In return, government ministers and senior officials then walk into those same corporate boardrooms – with no embargoes from Acoba (Parliament's advisory committee on business appointments).
- These partnerships, greased by political donations and hospitality, infect the major political parties. It is difficult to distinguish between cabinets and boardrooms, and decide which is in control. Even MPs take 'second jobs' as corporate advocates inside Parliament. Surely being an MP is a full-time job.
- With dogma comes a refusal to review outcomes and recognize generic failure. Most privatized utilities are little better than the water monopolies, private equity care homes put profit before service quality, PFI schools and hospitals are in hoc to their contract holders (mostly banks and private investors), while privately-run GP surgeries are inferior.
- Most 'checks and balances' to government activity, like the civil service, the church and House of Lords, have all been sidelined. The media, the most important 'to hold truth to power', now puts profit and prejudice above investigative journalism and integrity. Rothermere, Barclays and Murdoch are themselves part of this incestuous government partnership.
- As description of Britain today, 'There is no such thing as society' is fairly accurate. Increasingly it has become prescription for strategy, as mega-corps managing public services extract excessive profits, and governments reduce taxes. Both seem indifferent to poverty and 'benefit scroungers', the homeless, disabled, ethnic minorities and, most shamefully, destitute refugees.
- Yet tax evasion (ipE) among the wealthy is widely unremarked. While plumbers will be fined or imprisoned for tax evasion of £50,000, the wealthy (including a few government ministers) can evade tax bills measured in £ millions.

Finally, after four decades of squeezing all public service finances (excepting the Blair and Brown governments), democracy finally struck. Ambulance drivers, doctors, nurses and paramedics, post and railway workers, bus drivers, lecturers and teachers have repeatedly gone on strike. The government lamely refuses to negotiate, arguing the need to reduce inflation. Yet it ignores the real drop in their wages and conditions, the excessive salary inflation of the high earners and the unjustified price increases by the foodsheds, oil companies and energy suppliers. Wages percolate through society like manure. When profits are privatized (or 'siphoned off'), then the 'trickle-down effect' is derisory, if not illusory.

In conclusion, we must revive the tripartite system that has developed since 1215. The Magna Carta established an uneasy relationship between king and barons, state and towns, with basic rights for citizens. By 1832, citizens (restricted to male property owners!) had the vote, while in 1848, comprehensive responsibilities for local councils and public health were defined in law. We must now reverse the current trickle-down of funding and responsibilities from central to local government, so that councils once more manage their areas and deliver proper public services. This would revive council standing, citizen interest and local democracy. At present, local elections, with the lowest turnouts in Europe, are treated by the media as little more than opinion polls for a general election.

To enforce the three tiers of government, we should also elevate the role of citizens. First, we can no longer deny the need for proportional representation, so that MPs more closely reflect the votes of each party.

And second, if central government decides national strategy and largely funds local councils to provide public services, might not citizens be given some basic controls over government. The House of Lords, long overdue for reform, should be replaced by a citizens' assembly, with 100 (?) citizens selected like juries, for three sessions a year as now, but with a new assembly for each session, rotating between say 15 cities, including the four UK capitals. As well as discussing proposed legislation as now, it might also commission Public Inquiries, approve National Audit reports and set parliamentary standards – at present, all wrongly controlled by government. The assembly might even set up independent regulators for the media, accountancy, banking and legal professions that, like the government, currently regulate themselves. 'Self-regulation' is an oxymoron.

Three strategies might indicate a party that is fit to govern. The first is Brexit. Until we address this disaster, if only by joining the customs union, even the most rudimentary employment, environmental and legal safeguards will be in jeopardy, quite apart from the economic damage.

The second trigger for real change would be a government that addresses the barriers that impede most young people: barriers to adequate health services, housing and fair rents, to universities, skills training and jobs with fair pay, and now even barriers to voting and protesting. The first government to tap into the alleged idealism of youth might also find its resolve to tackle global warming strengthened, which in turn might attract more young people to the political process.

And if youth can't trigger action to address this third crisis, and no one party is brave enough to implement 'the unpalatable', perhaps some form of coalition, or even national government, is needed if we are to curb our unsustainable behaviour and expectations.

Conclusion

The official Covid inquiry will focus on how well we managed the pandemic and define how to be better prepared in the future.

This inquiry is different. It looks at all aspects of public health, environmental, economic and social, not just the pandemic. It also addresses the EU challenge of how to emerge from Covid with a 'green' recovery programme that meets the urgent needs of global warming, a sustainable economy and a just society.

This will be difficult. Margaret Thatcher's assertion that "There is no such thing as society", half accurate as a description, is disastrous as a prescription for policy, denying our very nature as a social species. With society increasingly polarized between rich and poor, young and old, north and south, shops replaced by the web, cash by cards and now most banking, finance, energy, fashion, leisure, media, sport and transport each controlled by a few oligarchs, we may be entering a new Dark Age.

Since 1979, the ideology of unregulated capitalism, small government and naked greed is bankrupt, found wanting in efficiency and expertise, transparency and honesty, and worst of all, humanity and ethical values. 'Diversity built Britain'. Dogma as surely destroys it. Covid occasionally exposed these failings:

- the quality of public services is invariably reduced when outsourced to private sector profit-driven head-strong amateurs, as with the T&T programme;
- SMEs are more efficient, innovative and ethical than national and global mega-corps in providing necessary equipment and services. If small is beautiful, big is almost always bad;
- and scale applies equally to government. The more it controls public services and reduces local councils, the lower the quality of those services and the greater the threat to democracy.

To define a green strategy post-Covid, we should use the government's own five guiding principles for a sustainable future which, since at least 1979, all governments have largely ignored. Consider each principle.

To 'use sound science responsibly', we must have relevant, accurate and timely information. For most public services, including education, housing, health and transport, local statistics are usually most reliable. National statistics smooth over local variations. When, for example, the first national lockdown was relaxed, many regions still had high infection rates. Relaxing restrictions was positively dangerous.

To 'live within the planet's environmental limits', we must treat global warming as an emergency. During Covid we actually fuelled the crisis by reducing taxes on petrol and domestic flights, while increasing rail fares that were already the highest in Europe. And for decades, we have ignored road pollution that has been 'quietly' killing 40,000 people prematurely every year.

To 'achieve a sustainable economy', we must curb mega-corps and their global supply chains, and strengthen local economies with more local production of goods and services through SMEs, specialist clusters and local councils.

To 'ensure a strong, healthy and just society', we must reduce excessive health and wealth inequalities. The legacy of 'Thatcherism' is our indifference to homeless beggars, our shameful treatment of refugees, ethnic minorities and the disabled, and the emergence of ethical food banks, in contrast to our commercial banks.

And to 'promote good governance', we must strengthen the various bodies that could curb excessive government control, reform the House of Lords as one of those bodies to define parliamentary standards and remove the stench of corrupt political donations. We must also revive the democratic potential of local councils to deliver essential public services through their collective expertise and experience. For too long, councils have shrivelled under arrogant governments that believe they can better deliver those services. They can't, and their incompetence and corruption can no longer be ignored.

Nor can we ignore the catastrophic impact of Brexit on the business community, science and research facilities, on young people and our

Conclusion

international reputation. The sad truth is that, when sense prevails and we seek to re-enter the EU, our environmental, social and employment safeguards will have sunk so low that we will have serious difficulty in meeting EU standards.

But this book is essentially focussed on public health. Aside from critical health events like Covid, public health affects all aspects of life – personal well-being, a safe environment with clean air and water, economic resilience and fulfilling jobs, social cohesion, less poverty, fair government and more local control. I hope epidemiologists and public health professionals will forgive a planner encroaching on their disciplines, but in mitigation, planning and public health share the same Victorian roots in local government and the *Public Health Act* 1848. We must relearn how to think local, and to act local.

Finally, this agenda for a sustainable recovery strategy post-Covid, based on those five guiding principles, combines complex health, climate, economic, planning and political issues. To develop this strategy, the EU has helpfully added clarity. To achieve climate neutrality by 2050, it has 8 policy areas – clean energy, sustainable industry, building and renovation, farm and fork, eliminating pollution, sustainable mobility, biodiversity and sustainable finance.

It's time we started.

Index

Acts of Parliament
   Child Poverty 91
   Climate Change 37
   Health and Social Care 18, 19
   Housing 95
   Public Health 131
   Statistics 105
advertising 27, 123–124
agriculture 75–76
air ventilators 16–17
AT Medics 19
Attlee, C 125
austerity *see* Osborne, George
Australia 6, 11, 110
Austria 6, 17–18, 40–42
aviation 37–39

Bank of England 124
Bankers' Crash 9, 88, 97, 108, 124
Barcelona 11
BBC 20, 39, 105, 107
Bechtel (in Bolivia) 61
Beeching, Dr
   The Reshaping of British Railways 39
Belgium 6, 17–18, 40–42
'benefit scroungers' 52
Bester, Alfred
   Tiger! Tiger! 100
Bhopal 61
Bingham, Kate 12
Blair, Tony 86, 97, 105
Bolivia 35
BP 61
Braverman, Suella 107
Brazil 5, 7, 117

BRE (building research establishment) 62, 65
Brexit 7, 34, 76, 107, 108, 109–110, 128
British Gas 82
British Rail 39–43
Brown, Gordon 84, 97, 113
Brundtland 112
Buchanan, Colin
   Traffic in Towns 31–32, 39
building conservation 94–95
Burgos (Spain) 43
Burke, Edmund 112
business deregulation 108–109
Business Links 74
bus services 44–46

Callaghan, James 111
Cambridge science park 67–68
Cameron, David 108, 109, 113
Canada 17, 117
CAP (common agricultural policy) 75
Capita 14
car dependency 31, 35
carbon emissions 30
   domestic 93
care homes
   for children 89
   for the old 14, 21
Care Quality Commission 21
Carillion 62, 104, 114
Census 2011 103
Chamberlain, Joseph 75, 101, 125
chambers of trade and industry 75–76
Channel 4, 107
children at risk 89

ChilversMcCrea 20
China 6, 35, 55–56, 69, 107, 117
Circle Health Holdings 19
citizens' assembly 127–128
civil service 114–115
Coase, Ronald 59, 60
Community Renewal Fund 82–83
Companies House 104
Competition and Markets Authority 89
COP 26, 29
corporate reform 77, 108–109
The Corporation (documentary) 61
corporation tax 121
cost creep 37, 41, 124
Courts Translation Service 113
COVAX 13
Covid
    border controls 7
    and business 57–58
    political response 8–13, 103
    public messaging 10–11
    and schools 16–17
    and traffic 32–34
    victims 13–17, 80
    world overview 5–8
Covid Public Inquiry 1, 71–72, 107
Crowther-Hunt, Lord 114
Cuba 117
Cummings, Dominic 10, 86
cyclists 46–47

Dacre, Paul 106
Dark Age 64, 108, 129
Davies, Nick
    Flat Earth News 106
DBEIS (department of business, energy and industrial strategy) 30
Death on the Rock (documentary) 106
Debenhams 64
Deighton, Lord 68
Deloitte 114

Denmark 6, 7, 14, 17–18, 40–42, 57, 122
Desmond, Richard 96–97, 106
DfT (department for transport) 40
Didion, Joan
    Miami 70
disabled people 14–15
doctors *see* GP surgeries
drugs firms (pharmaceuticals) 24, 26, 60, 77
Duke of Westminster 121
DWP (department of work and pensions) 14–15, 83
Dyson, James 17, 122

East India Company 65
education 84–90
EEF (education endowment foundation) 88
'elective dictatorship' and democracy 125–126
electric vehicles 34–35
emergency services 36
empires 61
employment strategy 77
energy conservation 50–53, 82
Enron 62, 104, 114
Ensor, Sir Robert
    Oxford English History 115
ethnic minorities 15, 83, 103
EU
    Health at a Glance: Europe 2020 1, 17, 34, 57
    Euromonitor: *European Marketing Data & Statistics* 66, 75
Europe
    Covid comparisons 6–8
    health spend 17–18, 57
    obesity 45, 79
    rail traffic 40–44
    retail outlets 66
    tax/GDP ratios 117

Index

urban public transport 49
Evans, Harry 106
exercise Cygnus & Alice 9
ExxonMobil 53
EY (accounts) 114

Fairlie, JA
  Municipal Administration 73
Farage, Nigel 107
Finland 6, 40–42
Finsbury public health centre 26
Five principles for a sustainable future 1–2, 92–97, 130
food banks 82
Food and Environment Research Agency 113
Fox, Fiona 105
France 5, 9, 13, 17–18, 38, 40–42, 43–44, 75–76, 86, 117
freedom of speech/protection of truth 107–108
fuel tax excalator 36, 41, 48, 113
fuel poverty 82

Gaia 30
Galbraith, JK 48
Garnett, John 74
Gates, Bill 121
GDP 55–56, 57, 75, 81, 97, 109, 117
Germany 6, 17–18, 40–42, 46, 57, 75–76, 77, 109, 117, 121
GIAs (general improvement areas) 95
Gore, Al 53
Gove, Michael 86, 108
governance
  defined 101–102
  outcomes 125–128
  policies 113–117
  problems 103–108
  strategy 108–113
  taxation 117–125

government regulation 62–63, 108–109
GP surgeries 19–21, 22–27
Greater Manchester 12
Greece 6, 17–18, 40–42
Green, Philip 51, 120
Grenfell tower 109, 122
GSK (Glaxo) 60

Hancock, Matt 68, 69, 70, 105
Hanson, Baron 64
Harding, Dido 70
health
  definitions 5, 21–22, 26–27, 29, 56–57, 79–81
  inequality 91
Heathrow airport 38
HGVs 11, 43, 48, 63, 111
Hitler, Adolf 113
HMRC 114
Hobbes, Thomas 80
Hogg, Quentin (Lord Hailsham) 125
home insulation programmes 93–94
Home Office 83
household emissions 50–53
House of Lords reform 127–128
housing associations 96
housing strategy 91–97
HSE (health security agency) 86
HS2 43–44
Hunt, Jeremy 18, 23
Hutton Inquiry 107

ideologues 55, 70, 79, 101, 108, 129
ILEA (inner London education authority) 98
IMF (international monetary fund) 57, 58
income tax 64, 119–120
India 117
inheritance tax 121–122
InterCity 39, 48

IPCC (international panel on climate change) 30, 50
Ireland 6, 17–18, 40–42, 57, 117
Italy 6, 11, 17–18, 40–42, 75, 117

Jacobs, Jane
    Cities and the Wealth of Nations 67, 74
Japan 6, 7, 17, 47, 77, 81, 117
Jenrick, Robert 96
Johnson, Boris 13, 38–39, 105, 110–111
Joseph, Keith 18
junk food 23, 60, 100

Kant, Immanuel 101, 108
Keynes, John Maynard 81
key worker strikes 111–112, 127
Khan, Imran Ahmad 69
KPMG 114

Labour, Capital, Land 56, 64–65, 118–122
land and property taxes 121–122
Land Registry 104
Lansley, Andrew 18
Lawson, Nigel 69
Leicester 12
'levelling up' 82–83
Lewis, Michael
    The Fifth Risk 115
'Liberty, Equality, Fraternity' 81, 101, 125
Lineker, Gary 107
LLPs (limited liability partnerships) 104
local councils 11–12, 25–26, 48–50, 73–78, 97–99, 104, 115–117, 125, 129
Local Government Board 115
lockdowns 10, 32–34, 46–47
London, Smithfield market 43
LSCs (learning and skills councils) 74
LTNs (low traffic neighbourhoods) 35–36

Macmillan, Harold 79
Macron, President 12
Magna Carta 127
Major, John 36, 39, 113
Malik, K 89
market forces/social need 32, 77–78, 81–82, 92
markets – closed and open 66
Marmot Review on Health Equity 24, 91
Marples, Ernest 39
MATs (multi-academy trusts) 86, 88
McKinsey 114
Meddings, Richard 19
media moguls 52, 83, 105–108
mega-corps 58–65, 117, 126
Merkel, Chancellor 12, 83
Merseyrail 41–42
Mill, John Stuart 112
Milroy lecture 1976 24, 29
mixed economies 74–78
monopolies commission 62
moral judgement 101, 107–108
Morrisons 64
Murdoch, Rupert and *Sunday Times* 106

national curriculum 85, 98–99
National Forensic Laboratories 113
National Insurance (NI) 118, 121
National Planning Policy Framework: 2012 2, 94
NEETs ('not in education, employment or training') 90
Neil, Andrew 106
Netherlands 6, 8, 17–18, 31, 40–42, 47, 50, 57
new roads 37
newspapers, national and local 106
New Zealand 6, 7, 11, 81, 110, 117
NHS 9, 13, 17–21, 24–25, 111–112
Nightingale hospitals 12
Northern Ireland 110

Norway 6, 17–18, 40–42, 79

obesity and diabetes 26, 79, 100
OBR (office for budget responsibility) 57
OECD 17, 84, 87, 91
Ofsted 85–86, 89, 99
Ofwat regulator 62–63, 86
oligopolies 59
ONS (office for national statistics) 92, 103
Operose Health (Centene Corporation) 20
Osborne, George
   austerity 9, 14, 36, 97
   Brexit 109
   housing 96, 122
Oxford-AZ vaccine 12–13

Paris, and Baron Haussmann 31, 67
Pavlov, Ivan 29, 35
pedestrians 46–47
Pemberton, John 24
Perry, Ruth 86
Persimmon housebuilder (and Jeff Fairburn) 96
PFI (private finance initiative) 18, 86, 114
pharmaceutical companies *see* drugs
PHE (Public Health England) 9, 11, 18–19, 70–71
planning and public health 131
P&O 15
'politics of change' 95, 113
Pollock, Allyson: *NHS plc* 19–20
Popper, Karl 112
Portugal 6, 17–8, 40–42, 81
poverty 14, 82, 95
Powell, Enoch 15
PPE (personal protective equipment) 9, 16, 68–69
primary healthcare 14–16

private equity and retailers 63–64
private health services 19–21
private schools 86–87
private traffic 31–39
privatization 45, 61–63, 72–74, 89, 113
Probation Service 113
profit motive 58–65
property tax 121–122
proportional representation 127
PTEs (passenger transport executives) 48–49
public health strategy 21–27
public services 70–74
public transport 39–46
Public Works Loan Board 124
PwC 114

QE (quantitative easing) 124–125
Qineteq (DERA) 113
Qureshi, Dr M 9

Raab, Dominic 114
R&D, innovation and clusters 59, 66–67, 72–73
racism 83–84
Rae, Maggie (Faculty of public health) 11
rail fare escalator 41, 113
rail freight 42–43
Ramsay Health Care 19
Rashford, Marcus 16
RDAs (regional development agencies) 74, 75
'reciprocal altruism' 56, 101
Rees-Mogg, Jacob 109
refugees 83–84, 107
retail outlets 63–64, 66
Ricardo, David 99
road pollution 34–35
Rocialle Healthcare, Ayrshire 69
Rome, and Piazza del Popolo 31

Russia 5, 7, 11, 117

SAGE 10, 105
Salisbury (Novichok) 11
SATs (standard assessment tasks) 85–86
Scandinavia 7, 11, 81, 117
schools 16–17, 85–88
Serco 70–72
Sharp, Richard (BBC chairman) 107
Shell 123
Sherman Antitrust Act, 1890 77
SMEs (small and medium-sized enterprises) 65–69, 77, 129
Smith, Adam
    Wealth of Nations 56, 59, 65, 89
Soames, Rupert 72
social neighbourhoods 8, 31, 95
social platforms 107–108
South Korea 6, 7, 11, 17
Spain 6, 11, 17–18, 40–42, 117
Spire Healthcare plc 19
Stalin, Joe 113
stamp duty 96, 122
statutory sick pay 16
Sterne, Lawrence
    Tristram Shandy 80
Stiglitz, Joseph 89
suburbs 31, 94–95
Sunak, Rishi 36–37, 38, 95–96, 104, 110, 113
Sure Start family centres 84
sustainability 3, 55, 112–113
sustainable development 93–95
Sweden 6, 7, 11, 17–18, 40–42
Switzerland 6, 40–42

T&T (test & trace) 7, 11, 13, 70–72, 116, 129
tax 'evasion' 15, 104–105, 120–121
tax income 118–119
tax reform 117–125

tax spending 97–99
technology tax 121
Teesside freeport 74, 104
Tesco 59
Thames Water 62–63
Thatcher, Margaret 23, 44, 79–80, 105, 114, 116, 129
traffic reduction 36, 47 *see* also LTNs
trams and trolleybuses 46
Transport for London 42
Transport Research Laboratory 113
transport strategy 48–50
travel comparative costs and benefits 34, 37, 44
Treasury 90
    Budget, 2021 119
Trivers, R L *see* 'reciprocal altruism'

UK 5, 6–7, 11, 17–18, 40–42, 81
UKIP 103
UK Statistics Authority 105
ultra vires 116
Universal Credit 14, 81
universities 89–90
Unwin, Dr D (Southport GP) 26
urban intensification 31, 95
US 5, 7, 17, 21, 58, 81, 107, 117

VAT 8, 94, 123–124
'Victorian values' 34, 83–84, 100, 116
'virtual time savings' for transport 37, 44
von Hayek, Friedrich 59
VRT or luxury tax 123–124

wastewater (to track infections) 11
water companies 61, 62–63, 108–109
wealth inequality 80–84, 120–122
welfare benefits 25
    'benefit scroungers' 52
WFH (working from home) 57
WHO 5, 9, 13, 17, 34, 79, 91

Wilkinson, R. & Pickett, K.
   The Spirit Level 81
Wilson, H. 125
'winter of discontent' 111–112

work ethic (and SMEs) 65–69
World Bank 58

young people 16–17, 89–90, 128

PETER LANG
PROMPT

Peter Lang Prompts offer our authors the opportunity to publish original research in small volumes that are shorter and more affordable than traditional academic monographs. With a faster production time, this concise model gives scholars the chance to publish time-sensitive research, open a forum for debate, and make an impact more quickly. Like all Peter Lang publications, Prompts are thoroughly peer reviewed and can even be included in series.

For further information, please contact:

Peter Lang Ltd,
International Academic Publishers,
Oxford, United Kingdom

To order, please contact our Customer Service Department:

orders@peterlang.com

Visit our website: www.peterlang.com

Prompts include:

Claudia Aburto Guzmán, *Poesía reciente de voces en diálogo con la ascendencia hispano-hablante en los Estados Unidos: Antología breve*. ISBN 978-1-4331-5207-8. 2020

Tywan Ajani, *Barriers to Rebuilding the African American Community: Understanding the Issues Facing Today's African Americans from a Social Work Perspective*. ISBN 978-1-4331-7681-4. 2020

Marcilio de Freitas and Marilene Corrêa da Silva Freitas, *The Future of Amazonia in Brazil: A Worldwide Tragedy*. ISBN 978-1-4331-7793-4. 2020

Janet Farrell Leontiou, *The Doctor Still Knows Best: How Medical Culture Is Still Marked by Paternalism*. Health Communication, vol. 15. ISBN 978-1-4331-7322-6. 2020

Clare Gorman (ed.), *Miss-representation: Women, Literature, Sex and Culture*. ISBN 978-1-78874-586-4. 2020

Eva Marín Hlynsdóttir. *Gender in Organizations: The Icelandic Female Council Manager*. ISBN 978-1-4331-7729-3. 2020

Micol Kates, *Towards a Vegan-Based Ethic: Dismantling Neo-Colonial Hierarchy Through an Ethic of Lovingkindness*. ISBN 978-1-4331-7797-2. 2020

Josiane Ranguin, *Mediating the Windrush Children: Caryl Phillips and Horace Ové*. ISBN 978-1-4331-7424-7. 2020

Dylan Scudder, *Coffee and Conflict in Colombia: Part of the Pentalemma Series on Managing Global Dilemmas*. ISBN 978-1-4331-7568-8. 2020

Dylan Scudder, *Conflict Minerals in the Democratic Republic of Congo: Part of the Pentalemma Series on Managing Global Dilemmas*. ISBN 978-1-4331-7561-9. 2020

Dylan Scudder, *Mining Conflict in the Philippines: Part of the Pentalemma Series on Managing Global Dilemmas*. ISBN 978-1-4331-7632-6. 2020

Dylan Scudder, *Multi-Hazard Disaster in Japan: Part of the Pentalemma Series on Managing Global Dilemmas*. ISBN 978-1-4331-7530-5. 2020

Shai Tubali, *Cosmos and Camus: Science Fiction Film and the Absurd*. ISBN 978-1-78997-664-9. 2020

Angela Williams, *Hip Hop Harem: Women, Rap and Representation in the Middle East*. ISBN 978-1-4331-7295-3. 2020

Ivan Zhavoronkov (trans.), *The Socio-Cultural and Philosophical Origins of Science* by Anatoly Nazirov. ISBN 978-1-4331-7228-1. 2020

Peter Raina, *Heinrich von Kleist Poems*. ISBN 978-1-80079-043-8. 2020

Geanneti Tavares Salomon, *Fashion and Irony in* Dom Casmurro. ISBN 978-1-78997-972-5. 2021

Peter Raina, *Doris Lessing: A Life Behind the Scenes*. ISBN 978-1-80079-183-1. 2021

Matt Qvortrup, *Winners and Losers: Which Countries Are Successful and Why?* ISBN 978-1-80079-405-4. 2021

William Robert Adamson, *Mine Own Familiar Friend: The Relationship between Gerard Hopkins and Robert Bridges*. ISBN 978-1-80079-485-6. 2021

Robin Burgess, *Francesco Algarotti: An Essay on the Opera (Saggio sopra l'opera in musica)*. ISBN 978-1-80079-505-1. 2021

Guy Merchant, *Cathy Burnett, Jeannie Bulman and Emma Rogers, Stacking Stories: Exploring the Hinterland of Education*. ISBN 978-1-80079-686-7. 2022

Alena Kusá, Tomáš Fašiang and Daniela Kollárová, *Retail Marketing Communication and the Consumer Behaviour of Selected Generations*. ISBN 978-1-80079-855-7. 2022

Marco Micone (translated and with a preface by Beatrice Guenther), *The Enchanted Figtree*. ISBN 978-1-80079-813-7. 2022

Brian Arkins, *The Poetry of Sex: From Sappho to Carol Ann Duffy*. ISBN 978-1-80374-108-6. 2023

David Williams, *Covid – an Alternative Inquiry: Putting Health at the Heart of a Green Recovery*. ISBN 978-1-80374-284-7. 2023

www.ingramcontent.com/pod-product-compliance
Ingram Content Group UK Ltd.
Pitfield, Milton Keynes, MK11 3LW, UK
UKHW021822140426
5217IPUK00003B/37